Refined

by

Wanda Strange

PublishAmerica
Baltimore

© 2007 by Wanda Strange.
All rights reserved. No part of this book may be reproduced, stored in a retrieval system or transmitted in any form or by any means without the prior written permission of the publishers, except by a reviewer who may quote brief passages in a review to be printed in a newspaper, magazine or journal.

First printing

ISBN: 1-4241-7700-6
PUBLISHED BY PUBLISHAMERICA, LLLP
www.publishamerica.com
Baltimore

Printed in the United States of America

This book is dedicated…

…to God. Without His sustaining grace there would be no story, even more there would not be life. It is my hope and prayer that this story will point always to Him. This story is a remembrance of how God's grace has sustained me, personally and us as a family.

…to Ginger, whose child-like faith inspired me every step of the way. This is her story. Surviving cancer has made her the woman she is today. She has character born of adversity. I am proud to call her my daughter.

…to Kerry, my life partner, my spouse, my support, my love. Without his support I could not have accomplished any of my life goals.

…to my sisters, Lisa Bell and Patty Smith. Thank you for always believing in me, listening to me and loving me.

…to Barbara Crawford: You were the representative of God's presence every day of our crisis.

…to the family of believers. You were and are an extension of God's love in this world.

…to each of you, who extended yourself to us, thank you. You are much more than friends, you were and are family.

Acknowledgments

I gratefully acknowledge the patients who allow me to be a part of their lives, those who share with courage their struggle to survive and to thrive.

Thank you to those amazing caregivers whose courage and stamina push their loved ones to get through the treatment and make every day of life count. They keep the schedules, provide transportation, and monitor medications… The task is daunting—you are my heroes!

Thank you to my co-workers, the professionals at Sammons Cancer Center, Dallas, Texas, who encouraged me to tell my story.

Thank you to Martha Gilmore and Jan Aldredge-Clanton, who were the first to read the manuscript and affirmed my desire to see it in book form. You are mentors and role models in so many ways.

Thank you to Dan and Marilyn Griffin. You are an integral part of our story. As our spiritual shepherd, you helped us to walk through those dark days. I am so pleased that you are able to celebrate with us God's miraculous power.

Foreword
by Dr. Dan L. Griffin

When you add God to the instinctive life force of a ten-year-old, blue-eyed blonde angel, you have a miracle-making formula! Put in her corner two devoted, stop-at-nothing parents, and you will see mountains move!

Ginger Strange had all this going for her when the doctors told her she had a malignant brain tumor. But having strong support and faith gets you only to the beginning of the struggle. This story will grip your soul. As their pastor, I lived through much of it with this amazingly tightknit family. I knew the parameters of their marathon of hospitals, surgeries, and recovery, and still my eyes went moist in nearly every chapter.

When medical authorities lay the C-word on you, every cell in your body tightens. Ginger's little-girl faith buoyed her parents' confidence. The fact that Ginger's mom is a registered nurse only intensified her anxiety because she knew what they were dealing with.

This breakthrough tale of victory through faith and effort will encourage anyone in a similar situation. Wanda, story weaver and eyewitness of the drama, describes for the reader the often unexplained facets of how one resumes a life put on hold. We empathize, thanks to Wanda, with Ginger's reaction to the gawking stares of the discourteous when one is permanently bald as a teenager.

Refined is more than a heart-squeezing look at a child facing a bully of a disease. It is the diary of a mother's worst fears, a no-holds-barred triptych of tough love, nothing less than a manual of how to face the unthinkable without blinking. It is a feast of survival for those hungry for hope.

On nearly every page, the author credits the part played by her tenacious faith that God was not going to let her daughter die. It is full of weeping, laughter, suffering, celebrations, and family unity. Every parent of children, sick or well, should absorb this story until it is a part of them.

Preface

From ancient time gold has been used to produce objects of beauty and worth. The ancients adorned themselves and their homes with precious metals designed by skilled craftsmen. Since early times gold has been a medium of monetary exchange among the nations of the world. In the modern world gold has many uses beyond its value as the monetary standard. In addition to being the source for jewelry and objects of art, gold is used today in electronic applications, the aircraft-aerospace industry, and medical, dental and chemical fields. However, found in its raw form, it is neither beautiful nor useful. Before it can be fashioned into any object, gold must be refined to remove impurities. It must be molten then shaped. Both processes require intense heat.

No one in their right mind would ever sign up for purifying in the refiner's fire. We may pray with the Psalmist, "Search me…test me… see if there is any offensive way in me" (Psalm 139:23-4), not realizing that the testing of our faith comes from suffering. And because we live in a fallen world, we will experience it. Christ told us that in this world we will have trouble. Adversity—suffering—trials—these are the refining fires of our faith. As we endure and persevere through the refining process, God molds us into something of beauty, something that can be used to bring glory to him.

Refined is a story of God's refining work in the furnace of adversity. It is our family's story of His sustaining grace. Unlike the refining of a golden object, God's refining work is ongoing. He continues to work in all of us, His children, shaping our lives for use in His service. It is my prayer that you will be uplifted and strengthened by my story of hope and God's miraculous, sustaining power.

"See, I have refined you, though not as silver; I have tested you in the furnace of affliction."
—Isaiah 48: 10

Chapter 1

Preparing for the Worst
or
Get Ready, There's a Storm Coming

August 22, 1984 2:00 a.m.

    The house was dark except for the lamp on the table beside the chair where I was sitting. I had abandoned the nursing textbooks that were now on the floor beside me. I had spent the last several hours looking for a possible cause for the symptoms I was seeing in my ten-year-old daughter. Everything I read told me it was very serious. Still, I prayed that somehow I was wrong. I cried out to God "This could not be happening, not to Ginger, not to our family." Tomorrow was supposed to be her first day of middle school, and in an effort to hide the fear I was experiencing, we would get up in a few hours and I would take her and her friends to school, just as if nothing was wrong.
    The summer of 1984 had been a whirlwind of activity. But then, that was the norm for our lives. Ginger had gone to church camp, and we had taken a family vacation to the World's Fair in New Orleans. Unfortunately, all she and I saw of the World's Fair was the infirmary. The doctor at the fair diagnosed her with a stomach virus. I knew that something was wrong with my daughter, though I never imagined that it might be something serious. She had been having some episodes of headaches and of vomiting. After she had a day of being sick, then she would feel better and seem her perky self. I had taken her to the doctor three times that summer, if you count the doctor at the infirmary. Her pediatrician thought stress might be playing a role. My grandmother had died early that summer. Was it possible that she was picking up on my

sadness, perhaps taking clues from my depression? I knew that she was nervous about middle school. Could that really be causing all the symptoms?

Up until this afternoon, I could have bought those explanations. As I sat in her bedroom with her friends talking about their plans for the first day of school, I noticed that Ginger's eyes were crossing. The medical term is strabismus. After the girls left and Ginger and my husband, Kerry, had gone to sleep, I pulled down the nursing textbooks and saw the words that would keep me awake all night. I couldn't get my mind around the words "brain tumor." There had to be another explanation. I am a nurse, not a doctor. What do I know? Surely, this can't be. Still, somewhere deep inside, I did know that something was terribly wrong.

The nursing books held the cold hard facts, but in the darkness the facts were not what I needed. I knew that our family was about to face the biggest challenge of our lives. I also knew that I wasn't where I needed to be spiritually. I had been a Christian since I was a very young child. Intellectually I knew that God was my strength. However, I had never faced this kind of test. I reached for my Bible, and praying for God's guidance to give me the words I needed, I let it fall open. It fell open to a passage that became my prayer.

> "Create in me a pure heart, O God,
> And renew a steadfast spirit within me.
> Do not cast me from your presence
> Or take your Holy Spirit from me.
> Restore to me the joy of your salvation
> And grant me a willing spirit, to sustain me."
> –Psalm 51: 10-12

As I earnestly prayed these words, I felt a sense of God's presence and His love. There was no promise that everything would be okay. I was soon to have my worst fears confirmed. There was no promise that things would be easy. We were about to face the most difficult time in our lives. God's promise was that He would sustain us, that He would uphold us, and that He would be there with us through whatever decisions and circumstances we had to face. With this reassurance, I closed my eyes, still praying for a miracle, and I slept until we had to face the next day's events.

REFINED

August 23, 1984

    The morning started as planned. I dropped the girls off at school. I had told my husband, Kerry, that I suspected something was wrong with Ginger, but I had not shared the depth of my fears. I kept hoping that there was a simple explanation and that it was something that could be easily fixed. I went to my job as a nurse at an internist's office. I shared my observations with my employer, who helped me get an appointment that afternoon with an ophthalmologist in our building. I learned that there are definite advantages in knowing how to work the healthcare system. Somehow I struggled to maintain control of my emotions and waited until the end of the school day, when I picked Ginger up and brought her to the appointment. After an examination, the ophthalmologist said, "Mom, this isn't right," and proceeded to schedule a C.T. scan of her brain. By this time, I was really beginning to be frightened and called Kerry to meet us at Baylor.

    We waited for what seemed like a long time. I am sure the physicians were reviewing and discussing the scans. I am also sure they were delaying what could not have been easy news to deliver. These were doctors I saw on a daily basis and I trusted their judgment. They had known Ginger since she was a toddler. Baylor is not a pediatric center. They were seeing her because of our working relationship, and none of them wanted to tell us what was wrong. No one likes to hear bad news, and no one wants to deliver it. One of Ginger's memories of that day is hanging around outside the radiology reading room and hearing a doctor she had known most of her life, laughing and joking with one of the other doctors. She says that she just knew everything was all right; otherwise he wouldn't have been laughing. There is a lesson here for healthcare professionals. As a member of the profession, I understand how important it is to release stress. However, it is essential to be careful where, when and how having fun is perceived, being aware of the feelings of the patients and family members who may be able to overhear our conversations. Finally, after what seemed like forever, the doctor came out, sat down with us and told us that indeed Ginger did have a brain tumor.

At that moment many of the details went into a blur. Still other details are as clear as if it were yesterday. Ginger sat on my lap, tears streaming down her face. She was clearly in denial. Her first thoughts and words were, "There can't be anything wrong with my brain. I am too smart." We were allowed time to sit and process what we had just been told while arrangements were being made for Ginger to be admitted to Children's Medical Center, Dallas. We had been surrounded by all my medical support system, but once the arrangements were made, we were alone, just the three of us. We were left to cling to each other, numb, scared, and somehow knowing that our life was about to drastically change. We were beginning a journey that would change us as individuals and as a family unit. These changes would extend far beyond our little trio. Everyone who knew and loved us would be touched and changed by our experience.

My most vivid memory of August 23, 1984, came as we left the building. Ginger stopped us as we stood outside the Medical Towers. She had something important to say, and it was a defining moment as we began the fight for her life. "I will beat this. God is not through with me yet." How true these words proved to be! No, Ginger, God was not through with you then, and He isn't through with you now! It was the first time I realized the spiritual depth that my young daughter had. It was the first time that I learned she had lessons to teach me. It would not be the last time she showed me what complete trust in God's love is like. It would not be the last time that she taught me childlike faith and trust.

Chapter 2

What Next?
or
One Step at a Time

There is much to be said for the comfort of familiarity. However, we were about to be shaken from any comfort zone we might have known. I was very familiar with the Baylor Medical Center surroundings, but that was definitely not the best place for a child with Ginger's problem. We moved through the emergency room and the admission process at Children's Medical Center and the staff could not have been more wonderful. They are the best at what they do! We met the specialists and were told that she would need a shunt to relieve the pressure in her brain before they could attempt to remove the tumor. The shunt needed to be placed as soon as possible, and the procedure was scheduled for the next morning.

There were practical things that had to be addressed. I was supposed to drive carpool the next morning. Despite the fact that I was overwhelmed with my own fears, I was concerned about Ginger's circle of friends. The children had to be told and I wanted their parents to have the opportunity to tell them in a way that would be best for each of the children. Though her closest friends were deeply affected, they proved to be resilient, protective and unbelievably supportive. Kerry and I made a few calls from the hospital room, but it proved not to be the best idea. Each time we would start to make a call, we would break down into tears and our tears were upsetting Ginger. We made the decision that Kerry would go to the house, make the necessary phone calls and return to the hospital with a change of clothes and toiletries.

The day had been exhausting for Ginger and eventually she fell asleep. Kerry and I spent the night in the hospital room. My husband is a very straightforward, practical person. He prayed, asking God to take care of his daughter, trusting that the procedure would be done and that she would fully recover. There is a line in the movie *Steel Magnolias* that both Kerry and Ginger quote to me from time to time. "Mom, you worry too much. In fact, I never worry about anything, because I know you'll be worrying enough for both of us." The two of them tell me that I take on the worry quotient for the entire family. That night certainly was no exception. I don't remember much except being afraid and numb. Somehow we made it through the night. Morning came and we waited for surgery time.

One of the most precious sights we saw that morning was our pastor, Dan, and his wife, Marilyn. As they came into the room, they represented for me God's love in a tangible way. One of Ginger's symptoms had been double vision. Sunday afternoon she had said to me, "Mom, when we were in church today, I saw two Dans in the pulpit." When Dan talked to her, he said, "Two Dans must have filled up the whole front of the church." She laughed for the first time since we had gotten the results of the scan. Before the technicians came to take her to surgery, Dan talked to Ginger and prayed with her. He told her how he knew she must be really scared. He explained that we would not be able to go with her into surgery room, and how he understood that she was afraid to go into the operating room alone. He reminded her that there was nowhere she would ever go that God would not be with her. God would be there the entire time watching over her during surgery. He asked her to recall her scripture memorization.

> "Even though I walk through the valley of the shadow of death, I will fear no evil, for you are with me. Your rod and your staff, they comfort me" Psalm 23:4.

The emptiest feeling I have ever experienced was that morning as I watched my baby be taken into surgery and double doors closed separating me from her and taking her from my protection. It was indeed a false protection. There is nothing in life that prepares you for the illness of a child and the helplessness you feel. As parents you want to keep your children from harm, but this was a threat with which I had no weapons to fight. There was nothing to do but wait and pray.

I will always be grateful for the firm spiritual foundation that was given to my child. I could have never known what was ahead for our family, but somehow God had laid a foundation for all of us. Ginger had always shown a spiritual maturity far beyond her chronological age. During the summer she attended church camp and came back telling me things that challenged me to match her spiritual maturity. That year Ginger had participated in Bible drill, requiring her to memorize scripture. Since I had helped her with the memorization, I had learned them, and they were fresh in my memory. During the most difficult times, when I couldn't focus enough to read or to pray, the assurance I needed would come exactly when I needed it from those verses I had committed to memory. As we moved through surgery and through treatment, it became obvious to me that Ginger had indeed been paying attention in church. She had a lot to teach me.

Children are very literal in their understanding. They hear stories and apply them literally. Ginger came through surgery and was brought back to her room. To avoid nausea and vomiting, she was not allowed to have anything to eat or drink. She kept crying, saying that her throat hurt and that she was thirsty. She was begging for water. As I stood by her bed, she looked at me and said, "Mommy, can we pray?"

"Sure, do you want to pray or do you want me to say a prayer for you," I replied.

Without hesitation, she voiced her prayer. "Dear God, please give me your living water, like the woman at the well, so I will not be thirsty anymore." Almost immediately she quieted, fell restfully asleep and through four surgeries and multiple procedures, never experienced that kind of thirst again. Many of the difficult days of treatment are blocked from Ginger's memory. However, when she tells her own story, she remembers the details of this part of her story vividly. She will talk about how she had heard the story of the Samaritan woman at the well in Sunday school, and she had child-like faith that if she asked something of God, he would answer her.

Every day brought new experiences and new challenges. One of the more traumatic was the change in Ginger's appearance. Just a few weeks earlier she had gotten a stylish new shoulder-length haircut, a dramatic change from her previously long thick blond hair. She was told that they were going to shave her hair. Knowing that it will happen cannot prepare you for the reality of seeing it for the first time. Not only did they shave the entire right side of her head, her face was extremely swollen, her eyes were black and the temporary shunt created a lopsided appearance to her head. If I could have kept her from looking in the mirror, that would have been my choice. However, she was curious and really needed to know what she looked like. She had been pretty stoic up to that point, and I honestly cannot remember her exact words. The gist of her feelings was that she now looked like a monster and she did not want anyone to see her like this. My boss, the internist, came through with a priceless comment at this point. He walked in the room, took one look at her and told her he was bringing in the hair dye so she could look like a popular rock star. She most definitely had the haircut for it. She also had the attitude to match the style.

Her self-imposed isolation didn't last long. A few very close friends were allowed to visit her, but only after careful preparation so that they would not be shocked or frightened. Reality is seldom as bad as what children fear in their imaginations. The bond between them is so much stronger because of the experience and the months and years that followed. Most of her visitors were adults and that was okay with her. Being an only child, she was more comfortable in an adult world anyway.

The hospital room quickly filled with flowers, gifts and stuffed animals. Ginger received gifts and cards from friends and family and even people we hardly knew. One particular favorite of the nursing staff was the giant balloon and flower arrangement from Dr. Macho and staff. (Yes! That really is his name!) The first of the stuffed animals to arrive was named Clyde, the gorilla. He remained with Ginger through all of her treatment, through traumas of junior high and high school. He has even been to college. However, I think he skipped too many classes to earn a degree. But he hung out in the dorm and is the only consistent roommate Ginger's ever had. Cards, letters, food, and calls assured us of the love and support of friends and family. Ginger's room was a favorite place for the staff especially the interns and residents. There always seemed to be pizza and goodies in the room, much more than we could consume, and we enjoyed sharing. The diversion was welcome, giving us something to focus on other than why we were there. Ginger seemed to enjoy the students and residents a lot, and we had many conversations about which one was the cutest.

Among the difficult challenges with a sick child is boredom. Entertaining Ginger became a full-time job. Barbara, our dear friend and children's minister, in a stroke of brilliance, brought a surprise basket. In it were lots of individually wrapped gifts. Ginger was instructed to open one gift each day. Throughout her illness and recuperation Barbara kept the basket supplied. One day the gift might be a stick of gum. The next day's gift might be a miniature Cabbage Patch or Care Bear, some of which still reside in a printer's tray at Ginger's apartment. Having a surprise to look forward to every day, helped to focus on something positive. Other friends kept her supplied in music and movies; anything to keep her mind active and engaged. We did whatever it took to pass the time and keep our minds off where we were and why we were there.

The next step was the "cool down" period. The shunt had removed the pressure from Ginger's brain, and physically she was feeling much better. However, the underlying problem had not been addressed. We hoped and prayed that the tumor in her brain was benign but it still had to be removed. What the surgeons were calling a "cool down" period would be the torture time for us while we waited to learn exactly what lay ahead of us. It was determined that we could go home for a few days and return the following week for surgery. We were happy to be home but waited anxiously for the definitive surgery and the outcome.

Chapter 3

Home Away from Home

Friday, August 31, 1984

We returned to the hospital as instructed. The surgery was to be on Friday. There seemed to be some concern about Ginger's white blood count and an increased risk for infection. Kerry and I were surrounded by a large group of friends and family on that day. They took Ginger into the operating room as they had done the week before. She was much calmer this time. When we signed the consent for surgery the previous night, I had a feeling of utter dread as if something really wasn't right. The experience of the "closing door" was different this time and not so traumatic. Almost as if I had done this before, so I could do it again. We settled into the surgery waiting room for a long wait. We had been prepared for the full day. Less than one hour later, the door opened and the surgical team walked out and talked to us. They had made the decision to delay the surgery because of her white count. What did I feel? Disappointment? Relief? Anxiety? To this day, I really can not describe the feelings on that day, but I know that I am glad that the delay happened. People were praying for Ginger, there in the hospital and all over Dallas, probably all over Texas. It was as if God said:

"Not yet, not today, it isn't time."

Labor Day, September 1984

Kerry's favorite holiday is Labor Day. It is the male bonding time. Dove-hunting season opens this weekend. This was the first and only

Labor Day he hasn't spent shooting birds. But Labor Day 1984 would be different. We were gathered again at Children's Medical Center. Again we were surrounded by a large group of very close friends. On Sunday night, we had signed the same consent forms. This time a kind and compassionate anesthesiologist used an analogy that for me made sense and gave me a greater comfort level. She talked about the risk that you take every time you get in a car, but that you do it to get from Point A to Point B. The surgery was like that for Ginger. We had to take that risk to continue any chance of normalcy. They took her to surgery; the doors again closed behind her. We are old hat at this by now. Been here and done this. "See you later, Mom and Dad." We really are settled in for a long wait this time. Today there really are more friends here, since it is a holiday and work schedules allow them to be with us. The sense of dread that I experienced on Friday is no longer with me and I am convinced that things really are going to be okay.

After a very long day, the surgeons finally emerge from the operating room. Throughout the day we were kept informed by the surgical nurses that the surgery is going well. We are escorted to a conference room. Barbara accompanies us to the room. Neurosurgeons are not known to be "warm, fuzzy" types and ours was no exception. The cold hard facts are laid out. Ginger's tumor is identified as a medulloblastoma, a malignant type of tumor with a very poor prognosis. Less than 50% of children with her diagnosis would be living five years from diagnosis, and of those 50% not all would be tumor free. I am not sure how bad news can be softened, but they left us with very little hope. It was as if they had dropped a bomb, and left Barbara to deal with the spiritual impact of what we had just heard. We sat in stunned silence not knowing what to do next. Poor Barbara... Her first impulse was to ask us if we wanted to pray. Before I could form a response, Kerry did. He absolutely did not want to pray. He was angry. He had prayed and trusted God to make it all right and at this moment he felt betrayed and abandoned. There was a room full of friends outside that door. Neither of us could talk to any of them. They all left without seeing us and went to a friend's home to pray for our family. Despite the fact that we were surrounded by people who loved us and that we held onto each other, I have never before or since felt so alone in my life. I truly did feel abandoned and forsaken.

Just When You Thought It Couldn't Get Worse...

When we finally were allowed to see Ginger she was in the recovery room. Her little head was covered with a thick padded bandage. She was still pretty groggy by the time they took her to ICU. Fortunately, the ICU waiting room of a children's hospital is not an experience many parents share. It is a harsh dose of reality. You and everyone around you is experiencing raw, numbing pain and grief. Some will leave that area to take their children home; others will not. It is my firm belief that we are not intended to bury our children. It isn't supposed to be that way. As parents everything in you wants to keep your child safe and protected. Here we were, unable to do what parents are supposed to do. There are no tools or guidelines to help you through this experience. The phenomenon that happens in the ICU is an experience like no other. People who are barely holding it together themselves will reach out and strengthen those around them. While we sat waiting in the ICU waiting room, I looked up to see a familiar couple, friends, part of our church family coming through the door. They had spent hours in this same room waiting to be with their son. Their son, who was born nine months before Ginger, had died of heart disease at the age of five. They knew what it felt like to sit in this room waiting helplessly. They were on the other side of grief. When they said I know how you feel, they really did. It cannot have been easy for them to visit us in a room that held so many difficult memories for them. They really didn't have to say anything—no words were necessary. Just being there with us was all that was needed.

We were allowed to see Ginger in the ICU as often as we wanted, and one of us was with her all the time. A side of her personality that we had never seen began to emerge. She by nature tended to be introverted and had always been a very compliant child. When she began to wake up, she was thrashing around and tossing her head back and forth. Kerry was terrified that she would hit her head on the side of the bed and have to be taken back to surgery for bleeding or something worse. He would stand beside the bed and talk to her very forcefully, telling her to be still and calm down. At some point, she must have had enough, because she started to yell back at him "I am being still... Give me a break!" A phrase that she would continue to use and the nurses would pick up on. "Give me a break!" became the short term motto for the ICU. As hours turned into days, Ginger didn't seem to be responding appropriately. Among her memories of the ICU days is a story about Carrie. Now, Carrie was the little girl in the next ICU bed. Carrie was about three years old and had learned that if she disconnected certain tubes, she could have the nurses' undivided attention. Consequently, her name was called out quite often. Ginger was very disturbed and thought the nurses were addressing her by her father, Kerry's, name. She would yell, and *not quietly*, "Stop calling me Kerry. My name is Ginger." She did at this point provide some comic relief in the ICU.

The physicians thought that perhaps she was experiencing ICU psychosis, and that perhaps she would do better on the neuro-oncology unit. So, we were moved to a room on the neuro-oncology floor. Though physically she seemed to be doing pretty well, the inappropriate responses continued. I had scratches on my arms and chest from trying to restrain her. A normally quiet, introverted little girl, she would yell at the top of her lungs. What she yelled about had just enough reality to be amusing. I have already alluded to the fact that neurosurgeons aren't known to be warm, fuzzy types. But Ginger took her irritation at that fact to a whole new level. She would yell at the top of her lungs, "My doctor never smiles. There is plenty of time to smile. You come back here and smile at me!" The oncology nurses found this most amusing. Even the neurosurgery resident found it amusing. When it became necessary for her to have a spinal tap to evaluate the psychosis, this big, good-looking, young doctor scooped her up in his arms and carried her to the treatment room. During the entire procedure, he continued to tell her, "I'm smiling at you, Ginger." From that point on, he was one of her favorites. That night as Kerry and I stood on either side of her bed, wondering if our daughter would ever be the same, she gave us the ultimate in comic relief. She sat bolt upright in the bed and began to sing at the top of her lungs, "I am stuck on Band-aid, cause Band-aid's stuck on me!"

While we laughed that night, we really laughed through tears. We were concerned, and when we voiced the concerns to the surgeon, his response was that she was doing well, and if we wanted, he could show us children who were not doing well. I already knew he was not there to emotionally support us. His job was to cut out the tumor and I really wanted him to be proficient in that area. We would get our emotional and spiritual support elsewhere. It was that night that I experienced a spiritual breakthrough. As I stood by Ginger's bed, I wept and prayed. My prayer was:

> Dear God, I cannot do this. You entrusted this child to me, but she is yours. I trust you to take care of her and I give her back to you. I can watch her die, but I cannot watch her suffer this way.

Unknown to me at that time, a group of my friends were together praying for Kerry, Ginger and me, being very specific about our needs. Since I had slept very little since August 22, one of the specific needs that I had was for sleep. The other was that Ginger had taken almost no food or water. I lay down on the cot in the hospital room and fell asleep, slept through the night and woke the next morning more rested than I had been in weeks. In the room was a basket of fruit that someone had sent. When Ginger woke up that morning, she appeared more lucid. For the first time since surgery, she was calm and actually asked for something to eat. All she really wanted to eat were the grapes from a fruit basket in the room. When those were gone, Kerry and I began to discuss where in the area around the hospital we could get more grapes. While we were having this discussion, a visitor came to see us. She was a friend of a friend, someone we had never met. The gift she brought was a fruit basket, and on the top…a huge bunch of grapes. Many may think this was coincidence. But I choose to believe that God cares about even the little things in our lives. He loves me! Those grapes were a physical sign that He cared enough to fill our need with a cluster of grapes. I know that I never had any control in this situation. I sincerely believe that in my act of surrender, I opened the door to the blessing He always wanted me to have. Were all our struggles over? Not at all! Was the rest of this journey easy? Far from it! But that night was the beginning for me of living with a different focus, one I still struggle to maintain. Stay in the moment. Enjoy life. It is short and uncertain. Look for God's blessings in the little things. He loves us and he wants to give good things to us. Does that include the Snicker's bars that the nurses told Ginger would make her daddy fat? I think so. When I let go and let God be God, "I surrender, whatever it takes," I believe he wants to bless me with "whatever it takes."

The Treatment Plan

Finally the blood counts returned to normal and the psychosis cleared. If we thought things were going to be business as usual, that illusion didn't last long. Surgical removal was only the beginning of the treatment regimen. We had been told that almost all the tumor had been removed and what remained could be "melted" away with radiation. We had also been presented with information about research protocols. None of the three of us was on the same page, when it came to research. The plan as it was presented to us was that radiation was a necessity. The unknown in the equation was chemotherapy. If we chose to participate in a study she might or might not receive chemotherapy. My one uncertainty in this decision was the fear of how we would feel if the cancer recurred, and we had not done everything possible. This situation led to some of the soundest advice anyone has ever given me, advice that I have repeated to others on more than one occasion. During one of her daily visits Barbara listened to me agonize and then said, "Gather the best information you can. Make your decision based on that advice and then don't look back." Ultimately, after several long family discussions, we decided not to participate in the research trials.

I have been told that in times of crisis you have to hear the same information several times before it really sinks in and even then your understanding is limited by your past experiences. Naïve as we were, I am not sure that we could have prepared for the month that was to follow. We had met the doctor whose job it was to try to explain the plan to us. The radiation oncologist was the antithesis of the neurosurgeon. Warm and caring, never rushing, he answered every question we posed. He patiently explained all of the expected side-effects. It was his job to tell a ten-year-old girl that she was about to loose all of her beautiful blonde hair. It was his job to tell her parents that he wasn't sure what kind of long-term effects it would have on her intellect, her adult height, or her ability to have children. All of this information he delivered factually, never creating false hope. However, he was the first of the medical team to give us any glimmer of hope that we might have a future. He ended our consultation by telling Ginger that he thought "bald is beautiful."

We spent several weeks in the hospital. The surgery had affected Ginger's balance. The physical therapists worked with her to make sure that when we did go home, she would be able to walk and not get hurt. She improved daily. Friends, family and even the medical team began to refer to her as a miracle child. Cards, letters, and gifts continued to arrive wishing us well and assuring us of prayers for a miracle in Ginger's life. Finally, she was ready to go home and we would begin the radiation treatment that would get rid of the residual cancer cells.

Chapter 4

Home at Last

    We were ecstatic to be home. Everybody wanted to do something to make Ginger's life happier and her homecoming special. One of my friends actually came in and wallpapered her room. A group of Ginger's friends came over and decorated her room for her homecoming. We had begun a scrapbook to hold all of her cards. It soon became evident that one scrapbook wasn't going to be enough. The church youth group created a banner of get well wishes that was signed by almost everyone at the church. Friends brought in food so that we never had to worry about cooking. We seldom had a day when someone did not come to check on us. This routine had begun in the hospital and continued at home. The first few nights at home were difficult for me. I had been sleeping on a cot in the hospital room. Anytime Ginger moved, I was instantly awake and up to see what she needed. At home and in our separate bedrooms I would be awake listening for anything out of the ordinary. She still was not very stable with walking and I was afraid that she might try to get up and fall. It would be weeks before I could sleep through the night.

    It was time to establish a routine. Kerry went back to work. Ginger and I assumed the daily trips to St. Paul Hospital for radiation therapy. We made the schedule and started to push through the next seven weeks. We were to learn much over these weeks. Life lessons to be learned went far beyond basic skills needed to return to school on target, beyond the healing power of music, and beyond the endurance it took just to get through the treatments. Ginger and I would begin classes with a homebound teacher who would come almost every day for an hour. I became a home schooling parent out of necessity. School work had always come easily for Ginger, and she was a very good student. Her recovery included some very dismaying surprises. Her handwriting which had been on target for a fifth grade student now resembled a beginning writer. The multiplication facts, previously mastered, were no longer in her memory. In fact, simple math had to be re-mastered. We spent many hours at the kitchen table, sometimes just Ginger and I, or the two of us with her teacher, who became an integral part of our lives. Student and teacher quickly built a bond. More than one education session was interrupted by a session of regurgitation. If Ginger felt the need to visit the bathroom, she would give a prearranged signal and the lesson would stop until Ginger could return to the table. After each such session, the teacher would affirm her little student with the phrase, "Adversity builds character." One particularly difficult day, when Ginger returned to the table and received her affirmation, she responded, "I think I have enough character now. Can I please stop throwing up?"

The overwhelming side effect of radiation for Ginger was nausea and vomiting. She vomited every day for the seven weeks of treatment. It was so bad that she would experience anticipatory nausea just getting to the radiation facility. I was sure no one could survive eating so little and throwing up what little she did eat. To this day she can not stand the idea of eating Fruit Loops, her favorite cereal prior to treatment. She had little appetite and I was sure she was starving to death. By the end of treatment she weighed only 55 pounds. The side effect for me was that I gained weight. I would fix us a meal or a snack. I would proceed to eat mine and then consume what she didn't eat of hers. There is no rational explanation of why I might have thought this was helpful to her. Somehow, I guess I thought I would feel better if I ate something. I suppose it gives a whole new meaning to the term "comfort food."

Another very painful breakthrough occurred with the issue of her incessant vomiting. The longer we were into the treatment the harder it became for both of us. One particularly difficult afternoon, we sat in the bathroom floor and I washed her little face with a wet wash cloth. As she began to cry, she said to me, "Mommy, I have prayed and prayed to God to make me stop throwing up and He isn't listening to me." I reached for an answer to a problem I didn't understand myself. Answering in the simplest way I could, I told her that I believed with all my heart that God was not making her sick. I told her that the doctors were doing things to her brain that were not normal and that was making her throw up. If she could just be patient, it would be finished soon. The radiation treatments were to make sure the tumor did not come back. I was honest and told her that I didn't understand why God didn't just make it all go away. I wish I could say that she never threw up again. But it didn't happen that way. She continued to vomit every single day. We continued to struggle with the *why's* and what to do to make it better. As soon as the radiation was complete, the vomiting stopped.

Just to keep life interesting and in an effort to restore something normal and familiar, we decided to resume piano lessons. Ginger loved music, and though, like any kid, she really disliked practicing, she really enjoyed the lessons and the performing. It was determined that instead of going to the piano studio, her piano teacher would come to the house for lessons twice a week. We tried to set aside time to practice, though this was not a real priority. We found that the skills required for playing helped her to regain some of her coordination. Music was so much a routine part of her life, that in any form, it helped to restore normalcy and routine. We listened to a lot of music during the recovery time. It created a diversion and smoothed out some very rough times.

The issue of self-image was among the most difficult of challenges. Bald may be beautiful, but try convincing a ten-year-old of that—well, good luck! You really do expect it. The doctor has told you it will happen, but somehow you think just maybe she will be the one who will defy the odds. We hit the three-week mark into radiation treatment, the area of shaved hair had started to grow back, and a part of me starting to think, just maybe it won't happen. Just as I had convinced myself that we might be spared this side effect, overnight her hair was completely gone—all, that is, except a little shock of hair that had been covered by a piece of cheese cloth used to pad the cast and protect her neck from irritation. Ginger has an interesting, yet to be tested theory, that perhaps cheese cloth could prevent hair loss in radiation patients. This loss was probably the most devastating for her and for us. It was the outward evidence of the inward illness. The loss was compounded by the fact that her hair had been one of her most striking features, long and thick and blond. She was extremely opposed to wearing a wig. It wasn't her! She had dozens of caps and hats, most of which she couldn't wait to give away. Self-image is such a critical thing to a pre-teen girl and building self-esteem in a child who has obvious differences from her peers has been one of my greatest parenting challenges. I spent hours and hours telling her that she is beautiful inside and out. No matter how much she heard it from me, she just wasn't buying it. "Yeah, Mom, right! You have to say I'm beautiful— you're my mother!" It is difficult if not impossible to shield a child from cruel stares and comments. Most of all, I knew that I couldn't be with her all the time to protect her from hurtful, calloused remarks. So, I did the only thing I knew to do, I continued to emphasize the inner character that made her who she was and repeatedly told her how proud I was to be her mother.

Election Day, 1984

We found it helpful to celebrate milestones. Marking the target completion day on the calendar, we crossed off treatments daily. We weren't a particularly political family. However, the target day for completion of therapy happened to be election day, 1984, and it gave us an end point. Every Friday we celebrated the successful completion of a week of treatment. The celebration was generally something simple; perhaps a purchase of some kind or some specific place Ginger wanted to visit. Regardless of how either of us felt we made a point on Friday after her treatment to carry out the planned celebration. Ginger and I had a tradition of doing special mother-daughter events. Since she had been to plays, musicals, museums and restaurants at an early age, it was a challenge to come up with a really special treat that would be affordable. On the last day of treatment we planned every detail. We went to the polling location and voted, serving as her social studies lesson for the day. We went to St. Paul for her last treatment. Every day for the past seven weeks, we had driven past The Anatole Hotel in Dallas. For us it symbolized an expensive place that we would not ordinarily visit. We decided that on the last day of treatment we would dress up and go to the Anatole for ice cream. And we did it! We completed treatment! We dressed up! I have no idea what I wore, but I remember vividly what Ginger had on. Her daddy had bought her a jump suit for the first day of

REFINED

school that year. She had not worn it again since August 23. Cute and confident, she walked into the hotel and ordered the ice cream. Ate what she could of it and then had to visit the restroom to throw it up. This visit stands out as a highlight, and the Anatole still serves a symbol of survivorship for her and for me.

Chapter 5

Are We Done Yet?

The end of treatment is a red letter day of celebration. But despite the feelings of relief and excitement on completing this phase, this can be a very difficult time. A concept I have only recently begun to understand. The daily radiation treatments are over. Daily visits to the doctor are no longer necessary. There is the nagging question, is it gone? Did we do enough? What comes next? All these questions happened to us in a sort of vacuum. It would be several weeks before we would have another scan to tell us how successful the radiation had been, and another surgery would be necessary to remove the temporary shunt. For the next few weeks, we were on hold, to wait and to heal.

No one tells you about the emotions that you are going to feel immediately after treatment. For me there were days when I felt on top of the world. We were done with treatment, and Ginger was beginning to regain some strength. I could begin to feel as if things might get back to normal. On the other hand, there were extremely dark days. We had been so involved in treatment, that little time was left for reflection. Before August 23, I had been a very busy working mother with a demanding job, actively involved in community and church activities. Suddenly our world had changed, and now I wondered what I was supposed to do next, now that we weren't doing any active treatment. Would the cancer come back? When would Ginger be able to go back to school? How would she handle school and social situations? I would return to work when she returned to school, but I was an entirely different person. Where would I find the patience to deal with people who complain of what now seemed to be insignificant medical problems? At least they were insignificant compared to the problems we had faced, and I had little tolerance for whining. I was plagued with many questions that could only be answered by time and experience.

I recall one Sunday morning church service during this waiting period. Our church was a relatively traditional Baptist church, not known for "healing services." But this particular Sunday was an exception. Dan preached a sermon on God's healing power. During the alter call, there were many people who came forward for prayer and healing. Kerry had stayed at home with Ginger that morning, so there I was alone at the altar asking for healing. The obvious healing I pleaded for was for my child—that the tumor would be forever gone and that she would have a long and normal life. But more than healing for Ginger, I needed healing for myself. I desperately needed healing of the fear and anxiety that had taken up residence somewhere deep inside. Surrounded by several friends on our knees, we wept and prayed. When I left church that morning, a heavy burden had been lifted. I left with a new sense of empowerment. I knew there would still be anxiety-ridden days, but I also knew that I could trust God with my fears and worries, and that he would continue to hold me as he had throughout each crisis that we faced.

One of God's greatest gifts to us was the love and support of the community of faith. I would tell Ginger that she was an ecumenical project. She had many of the churches in the community praying for her throughout the diagnosis and treatment. One friend shared that she prayed for us by keeping our name on her refrigerator door. Each time she passed the door, she would breathe our name in prayer. In this way she said, "Dear God, I don't know what Ginger needs today, but you do. Meet her need today." I found it empowering and comforting to know that people were praying for us. The support we received was more than prayer alone. Needs were met on a daily basis. Friends cleaned the house before we came home from the hospital. Laundry was done; the lawn was cut. The pantry was filled. Meals were provided. Cards arrived daily. We were constantly assured of love and support. God's people were the visible evidence of His care for us. Words can never express our sincere appreciation for all the ways they upheld us during those dark days.

Being a "Type A" personality, the grinding halt to my previously breakneck pace of life was a challenge. However, the blessing of this slowed-down pace of life was that I had more time to spend in prayer and

Bible reading. One day as I was seeking guidance in the scripture, I read a verse that jumped off the page and grabbed my attention. I have tried unsuccessfully many times since to find the exact reference. I only remember that it appeared as a promise to me. The gist of the verse was that I would be blessed with grandchildren. Since Ginger is an only child, that pretty much said to me that she would survive to adulthood. Admittedly it was taken out of context, but it was a gift to me on that particular day. I have no idea what God has planned for the future, or whether children are a part of it, but I trust him to care for and supply all our needs and many of our desires.

Family life was a challenge. Kerry, Ginger and I had always been a tight threesome. For some reason, when she felt the worst, only I could take care of what she wanted. I was physically and emotionally exhausted. Kerry would try to relieve me and give me some time to myself, but if there was a crisis, only Mom could take care of it. He had always been the protector and more of a disciplinarian than I was. But really more importantly, the father-daughter dynamic was teasing, laughing and playing. One day after he had been particularly hurt by Ginger pushing him away, I had a revelation of sorts. She associated Dad with fun and playtime. She was hurting and sick and she really wanted to disassociate him from the pain. Approaching life that way helped us to deal with the new family dynamic in a healthy way. We formed an even stronger alliance. Communication can be very difficult during times of crisis, but it is absolutely essential. Statistics show that many marriages end in divorce after a serious illness or death of a child. Communication and commitment for us were the keys to staying together and remaining a strong couple as caregiver survivors. Important decisions were made as a family and we worked hard to keep all the communication lines flowing.

Throughout the surgery and treatment, Ginger had mercifully experienced very little physical pain. We spent mid-November quietly making plans for Thanksgiving, working diligently on home school projects, and thinking that the worst was behind us. We were jolted out of our temporary respite when shingles broke out along her scalp. The doctor's major concern was that it not spread to her eye. We were to learn that shingles in the eye can have quite serious and permanent consequences leading to blindness. I nervously watched as each lesion broke out, onto her forehead. The last lesion stopped in the eyebrow. Shingles added insult to injury. It wasn't enough that she was bald; now she had to deal with sores on her head as well, compounded by the allergic rash she developed to the first pain medicine prescribed. However, the cosmetic aspect was minor compared to the pain she experienced. In the initial stage I gave her enough pain medication to just let her sleep through the worst pain. But once the blisters healed and she wasn't in constant pain, the medication was no longer necessary. The type of pain she experienced was shockwave like and occurred occasionally and without warning. The worst episode occurred during our family Thanksgiving dinner when suddenly without warning a blood curdling scream of pain stopped our celebration until the pain could be resolved. Still we were hopeful and thankful. The pain improved over the next several weeks; she was feeling better and the shingles had not affected her eyes.

Christmas 1984

Christmas was coming and we could focus on something else besides medullo-blastoma and everything that diagnosis and treatment involved. We had always been a two paycheck family, and without my paycheck finances during this time were tight. Over the months of Ginger's illness money had arrived just in time to fill specific needs. Amazingly, God supplied our needs through anonymous gifts overwhelming us with gratitude. Fortunately, we had excellent insurance, so paying the medical bills was not the kind of economic burden that confronts many people facing such illness. There was food in the pantry and our basic needs were never threatened. Still, there was no ready cash available for Christmas gifts.

We were determined to make Christmas a celebration and carry out our family traditions. We hauled the decorations out of the attic and decorated the house. It is a tradition in our family that we fill the house with Christmas music and decorate not just the tree but the entire house together. This usually occurs in late November or early December, preferably the Friday or Saturday after Thanksgiving. I am of the opinion that decorating is too much work not to enjoy it for the entire month.

Christmas 1984, we desperately needed to focus on Christmas celebration and not the crisis that had dominated our daily existence. And so, we did all the familiar things that brought us comfort. We decorated. We baked Christmas cookies. Instead of singing in the Christmas choir programs as we usually did, we sat back and enjoyed listening to the music.

Our longest-standing tradition for Christmas had been helping with distribution of Christmas gifts and food to needy families. I started taking Ginger with me when she was a toddler. We were not and are not by any means a wealthy family, just a hard-working two-income middle-class family. We have always felt blessed. I was determined to model a caring, giving spirit for my child. As she is fond of saying, she may be spoiled but she is not undisciplined. She also has a tender heart. This year we would not be able to carry out this tradition. One of the worst parts of crisis is how it focuses your energies inward. The most valuable lesson for me was to allow others to minister to me. In early December a friend called to inquire about Ginger's sizes and to inform me that our Sunday school class would be handling Christmas gifts.

Christmas Eve arrived and so did the gifts. Not only did they bring gifts for Ginger, they filled our pantry with enough food to carry us through the next months. I was absolutely overwhelmed with emotion. They did for us what we could not do. Our Christmas would have been slim, but we would have still celebrated Jesus' birthday. The Christmas celebration had taken on a deeper meaning for all of us.

The outpouring of love and gifts from our friends was extravagant. There were so many gifts that it took the most of Christmas morning for her to open them. After breakfast, she put on a style show for us with all her new clothes, each ensemble completed by a matching hat. She had a wonderful time posing for pictures in each new outfit. There were more toys and games than she could play with in one day. Christmas 1985 was sure to be a come down. No gift had a name on it. No one wanted acknowledgement. They gave because they loved her and us. They gave as an expression and an extension of God's extravagant love. I had the only gift I wanted that day. I was surrounded by friends and family and I was able to cuddle with my child. I delighted in seeing her happiness. When any of the three of us is asked to describe our most memorable holiday, it is Christmas 1984—hands down.

REFINED

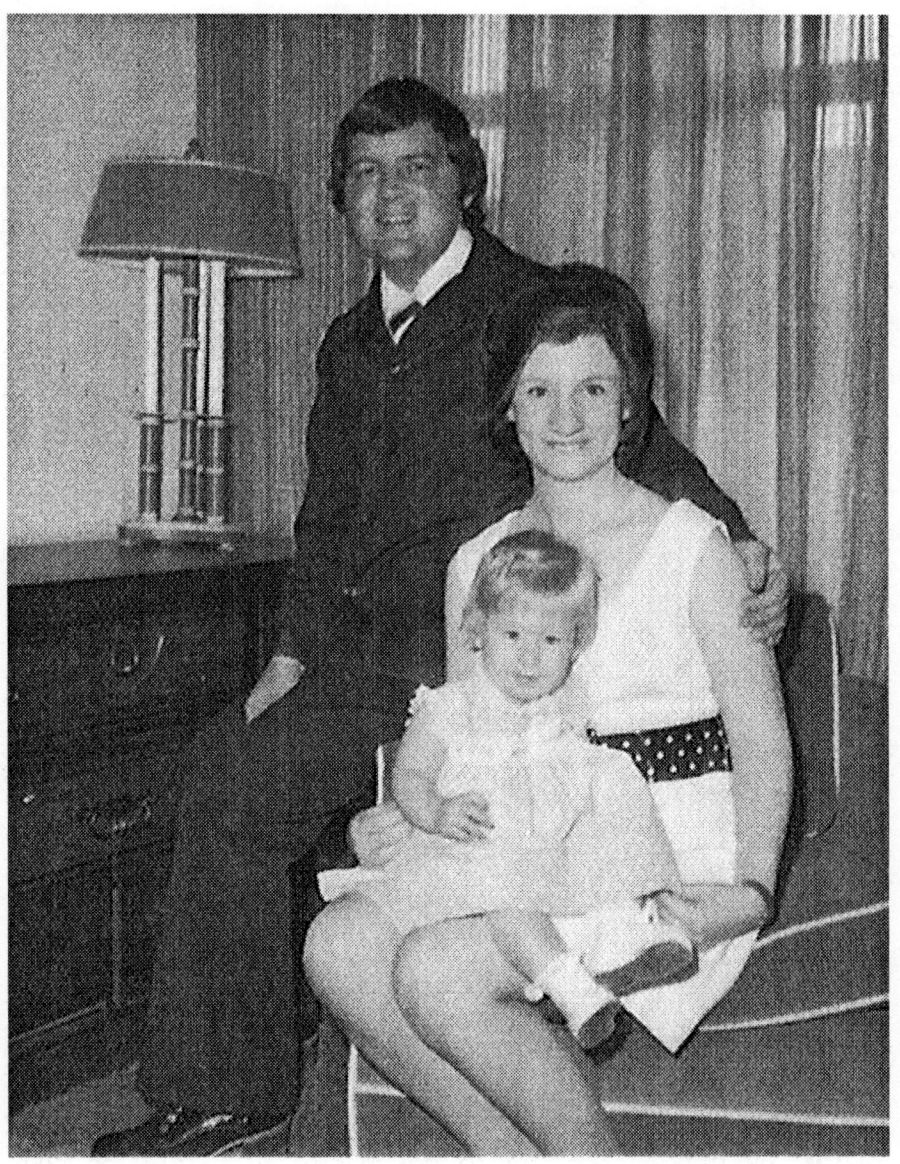

Dedication Day, May 1975

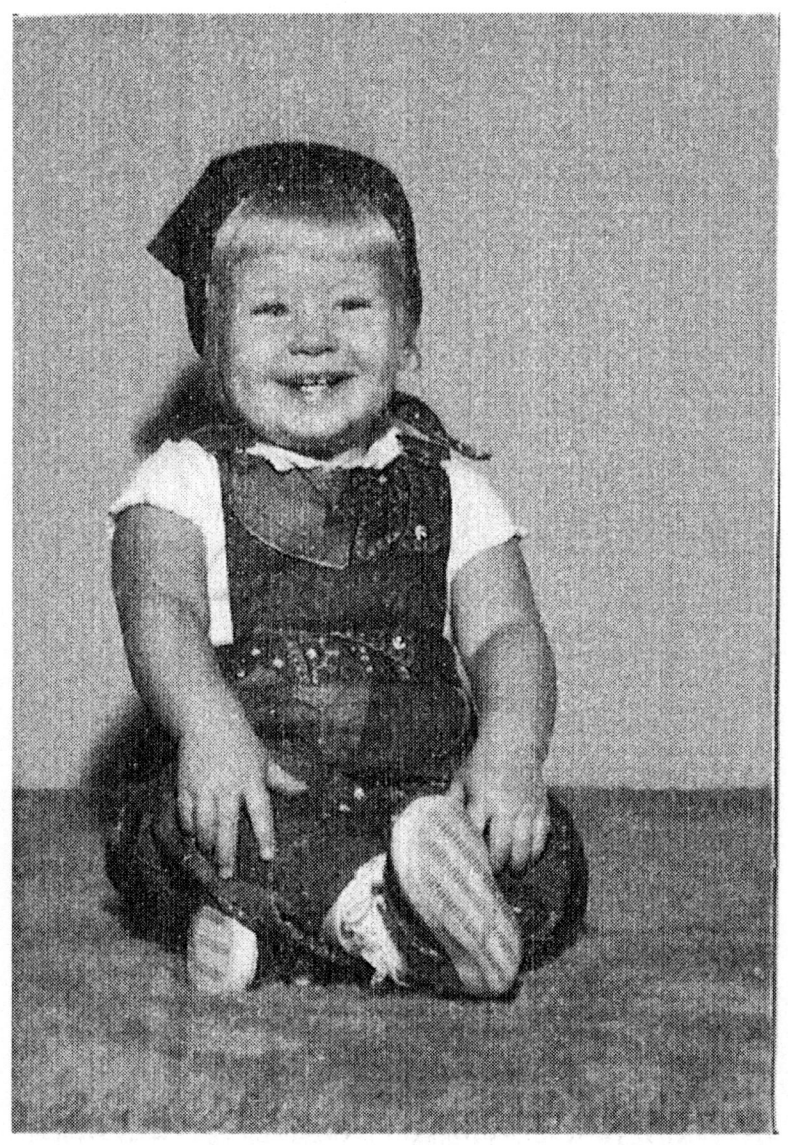

Dad's favorite Ginger picture—18 months

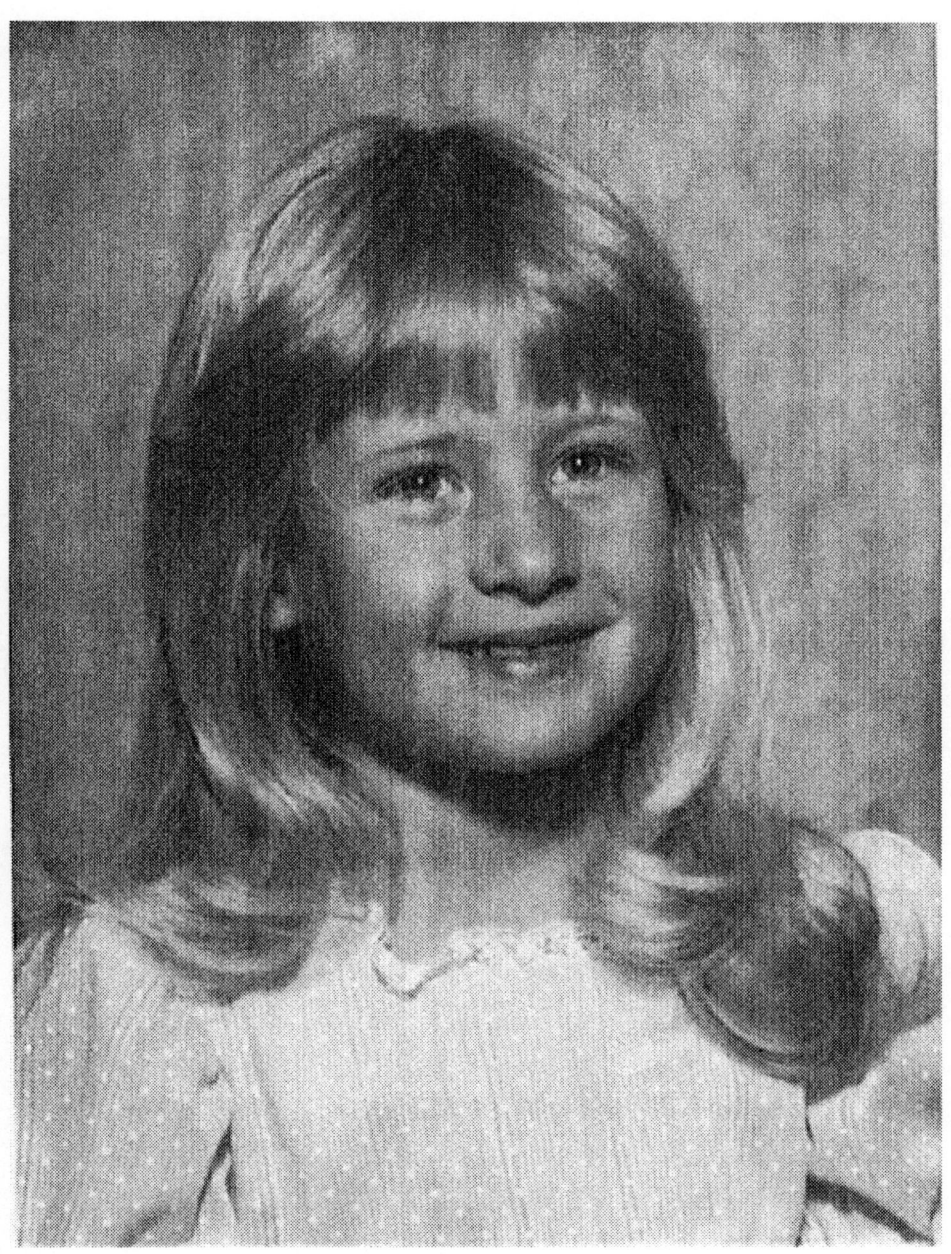

Ginger, age 5

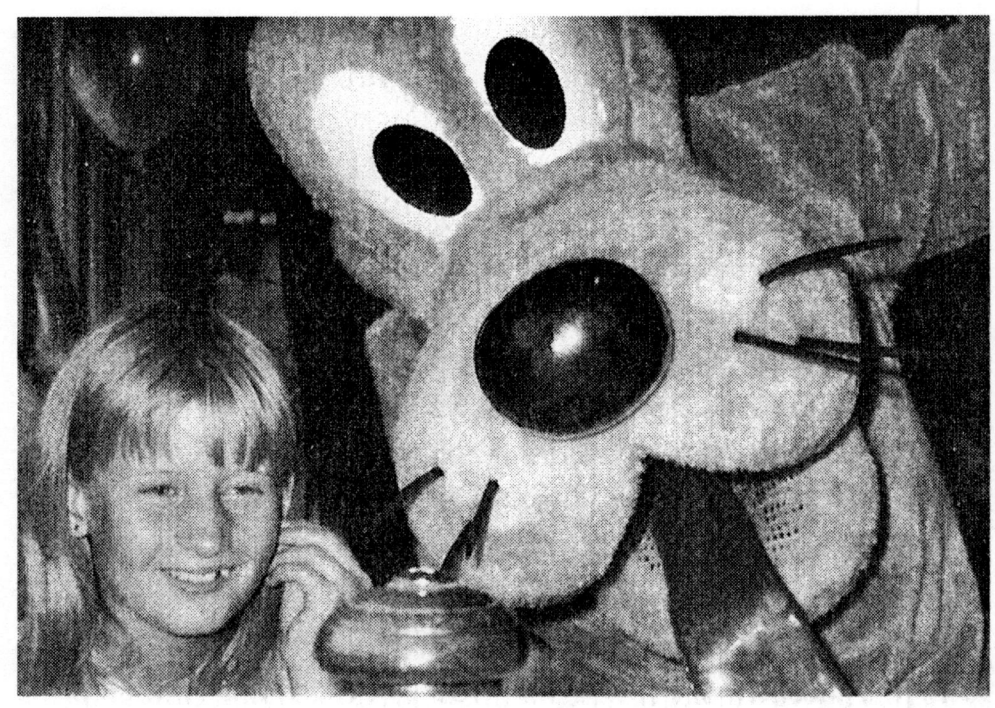

Ginger and Goofy at Disney World, 1982

REFINED

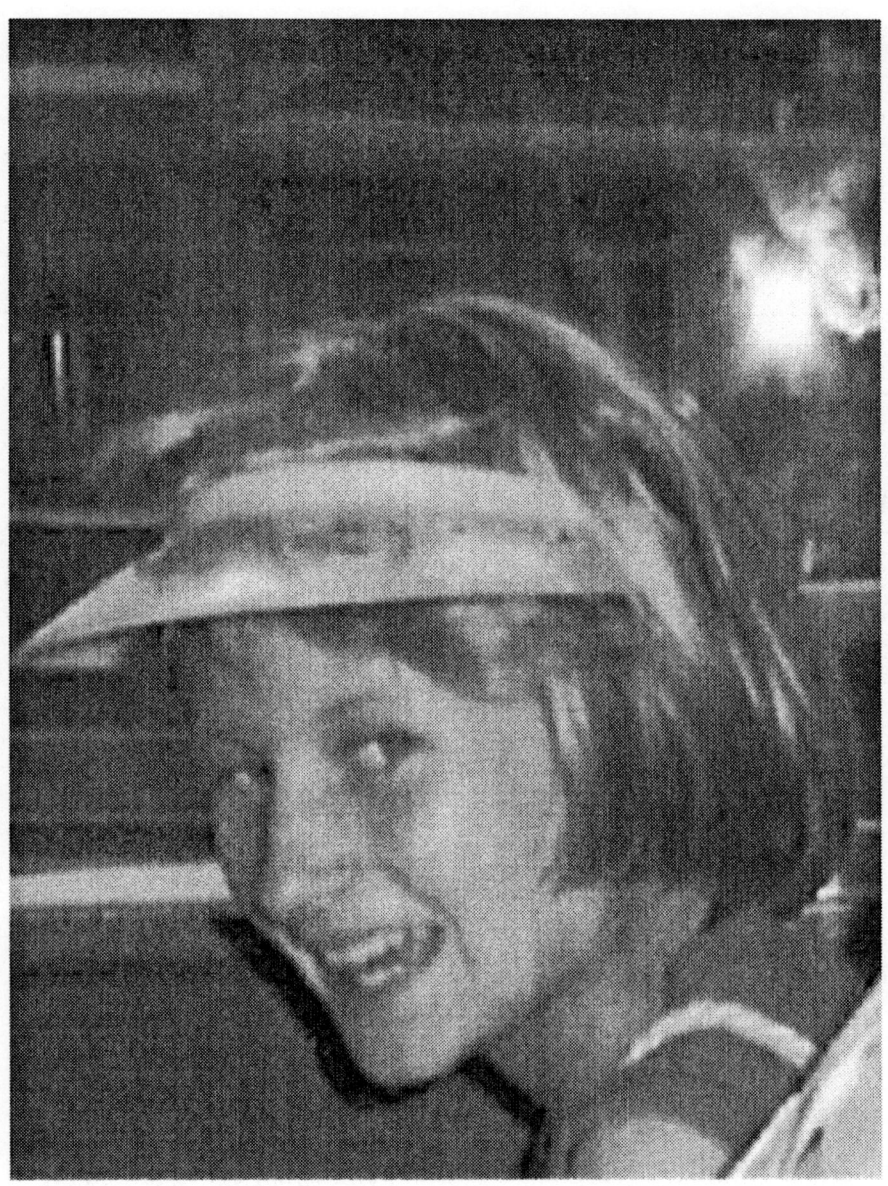

One month prior to diagnosis on a New Orleans Streetcar for the World's Fair

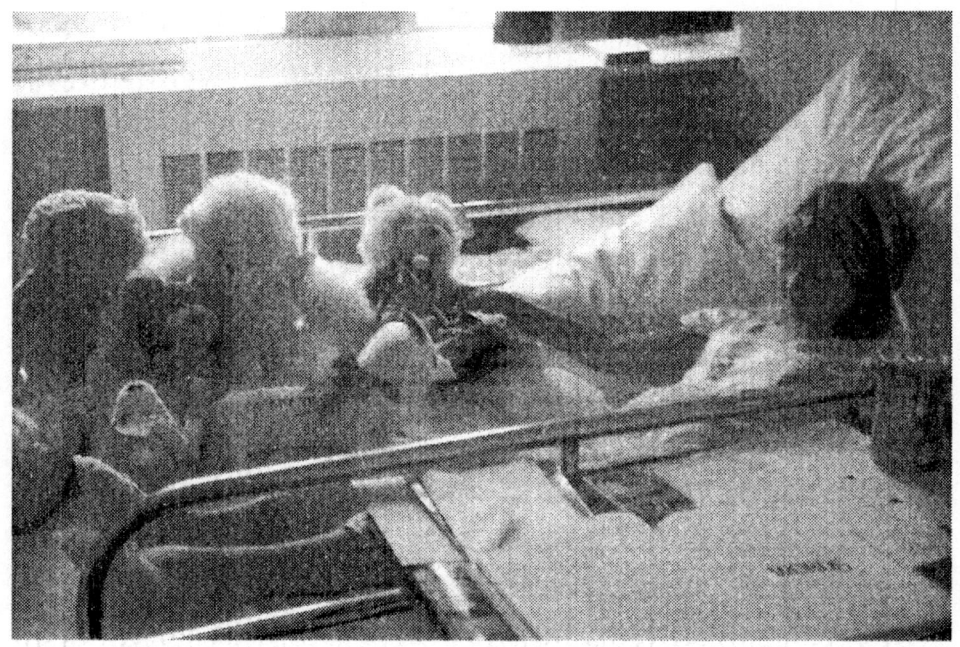

Ginger in the hospital after one of several surgeries

REFINED

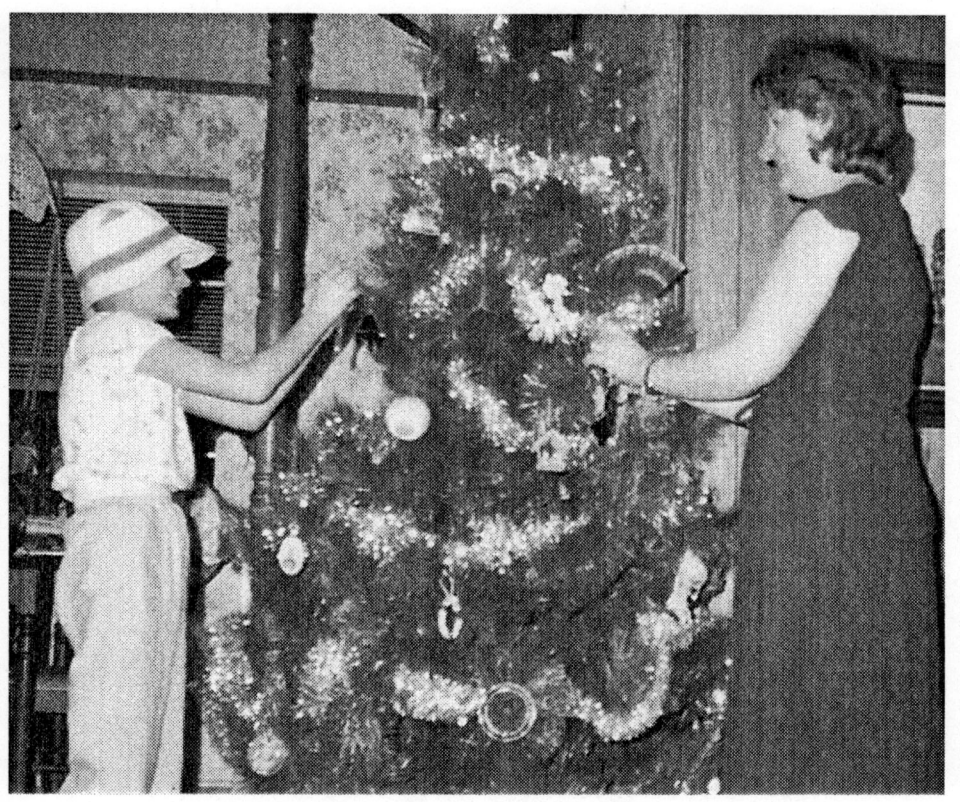

Decorating the Christmas tree, 1984

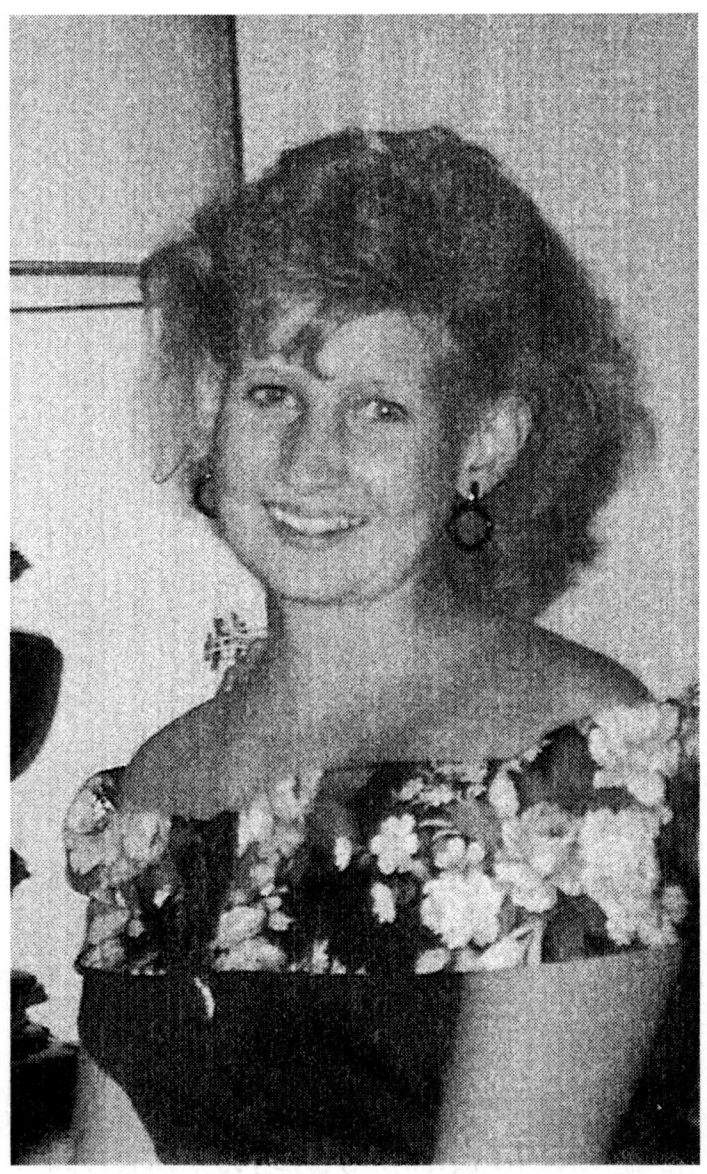

Ginger, age 15

REFINED

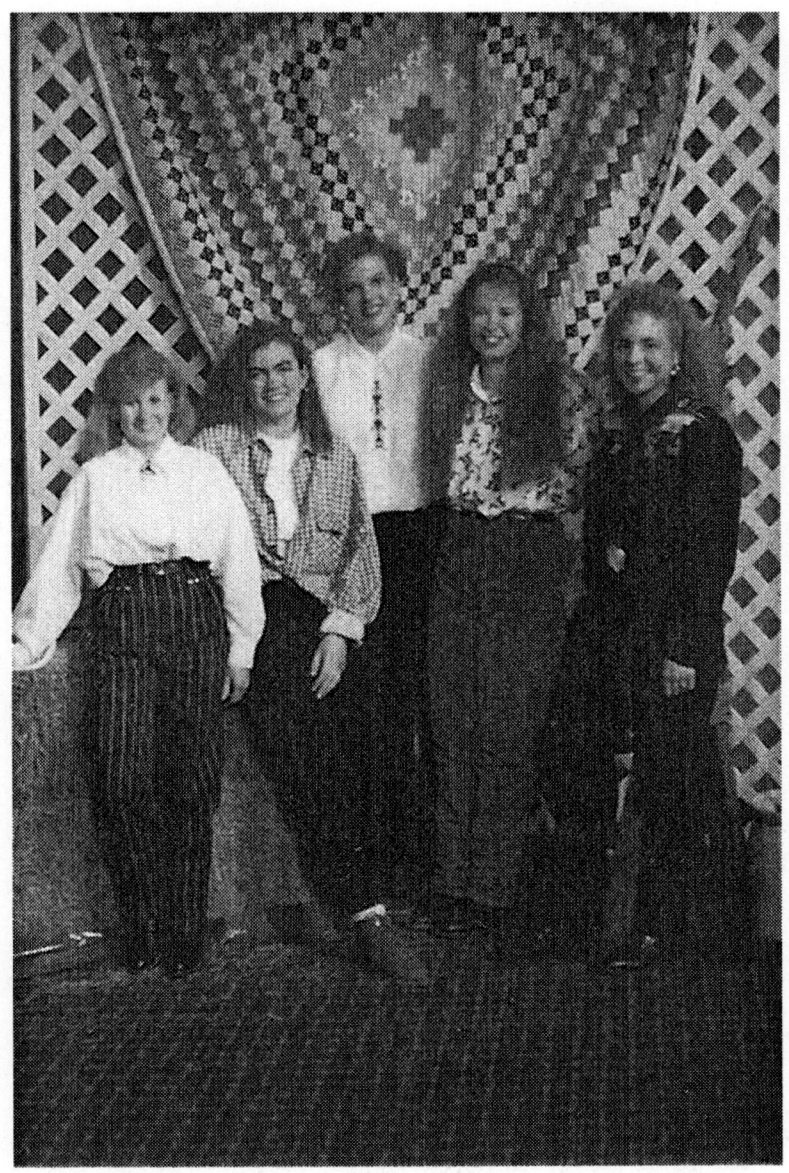

Ginger, Stephanie, Amy, Cristen, Amy
Surviving the difficult teen years together

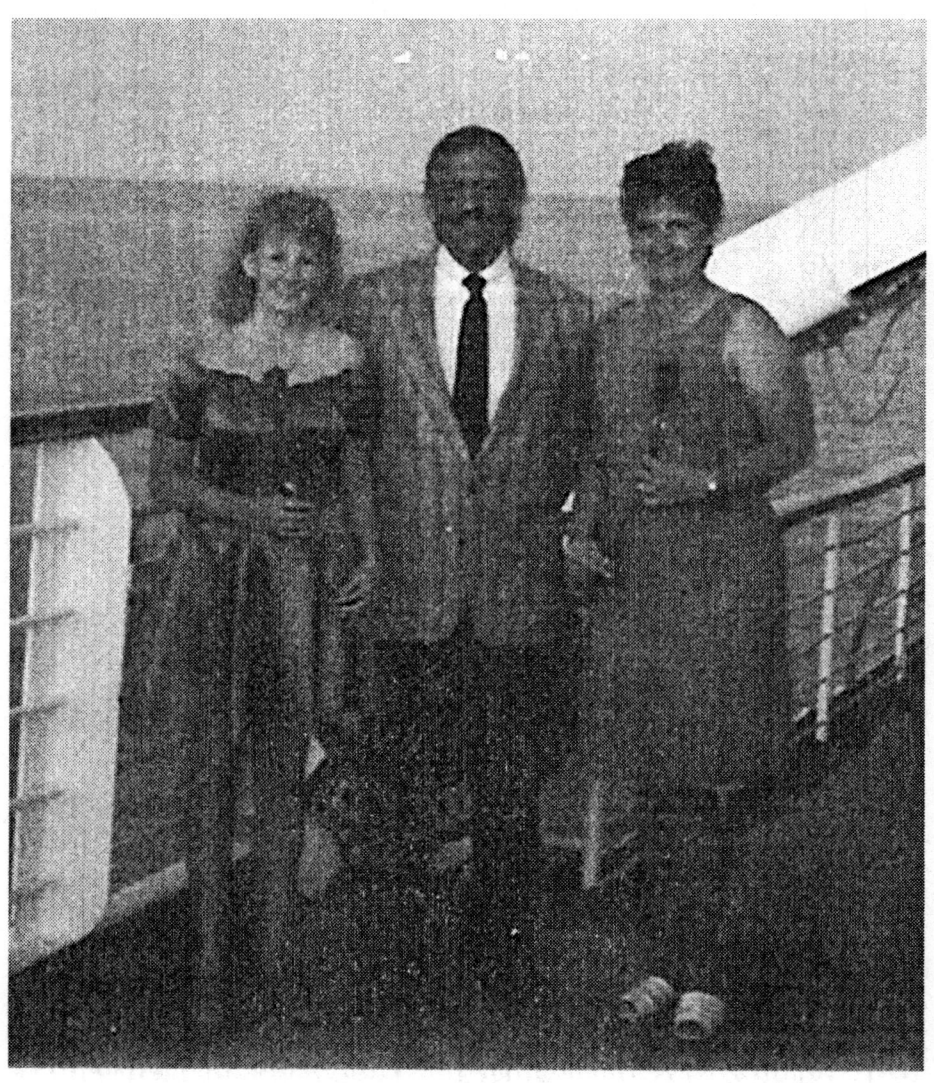

Cruising the Carribean to celebrate high school graduation

REFINED

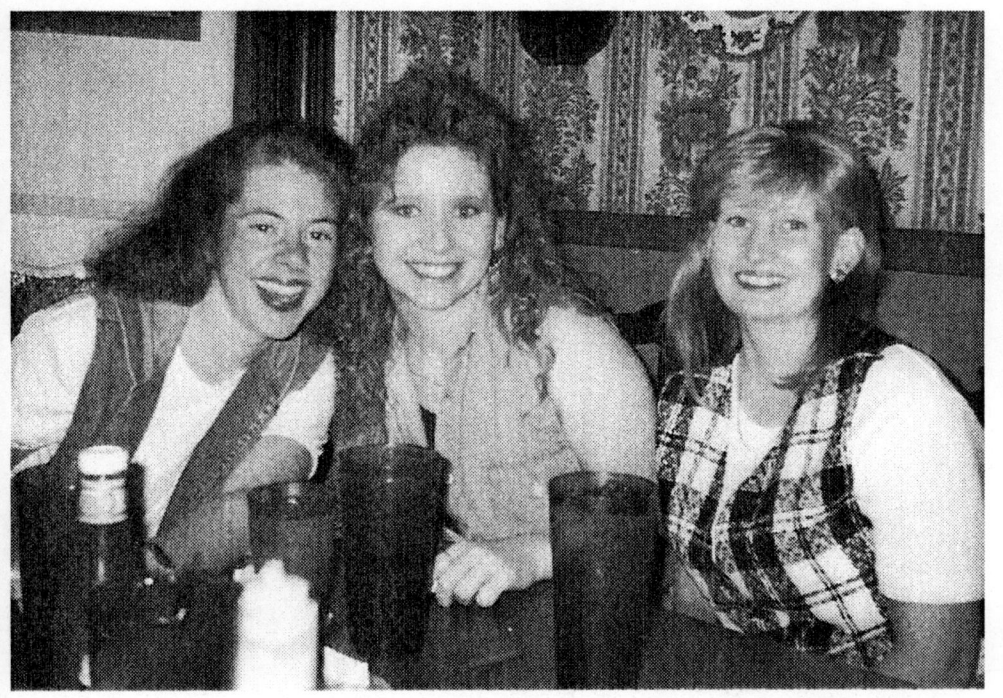

M'Lynne, Frankie, and Ginger, out to dinner during the college days

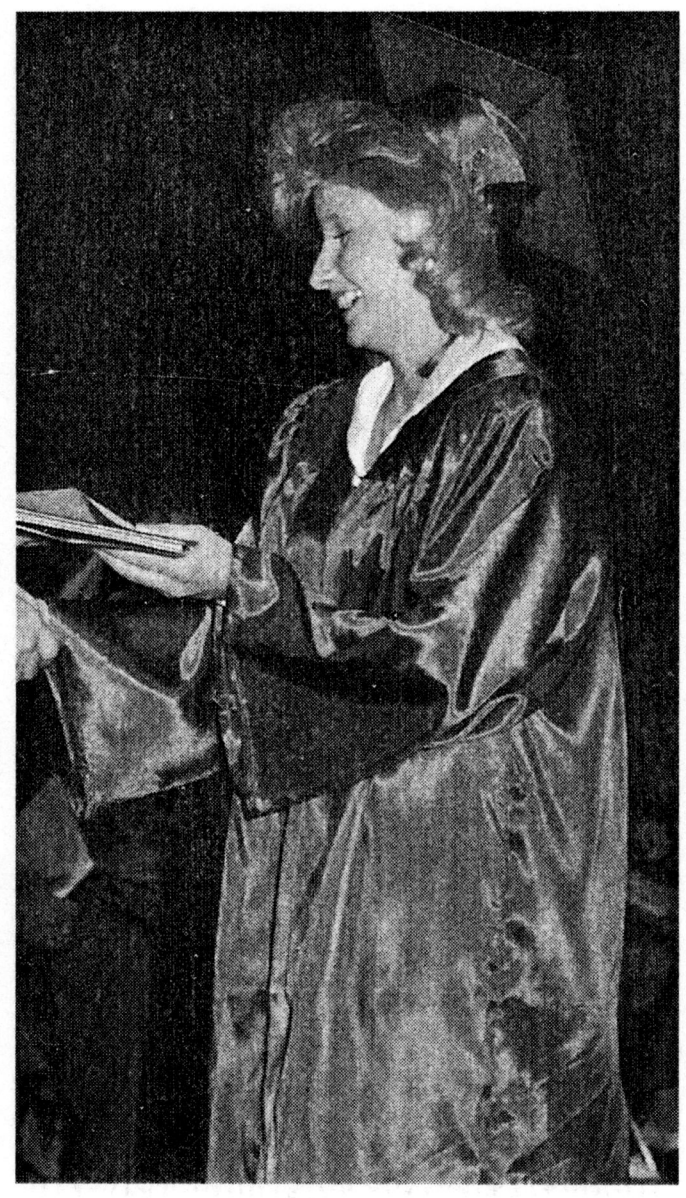

Graduation from West Texas A&M University

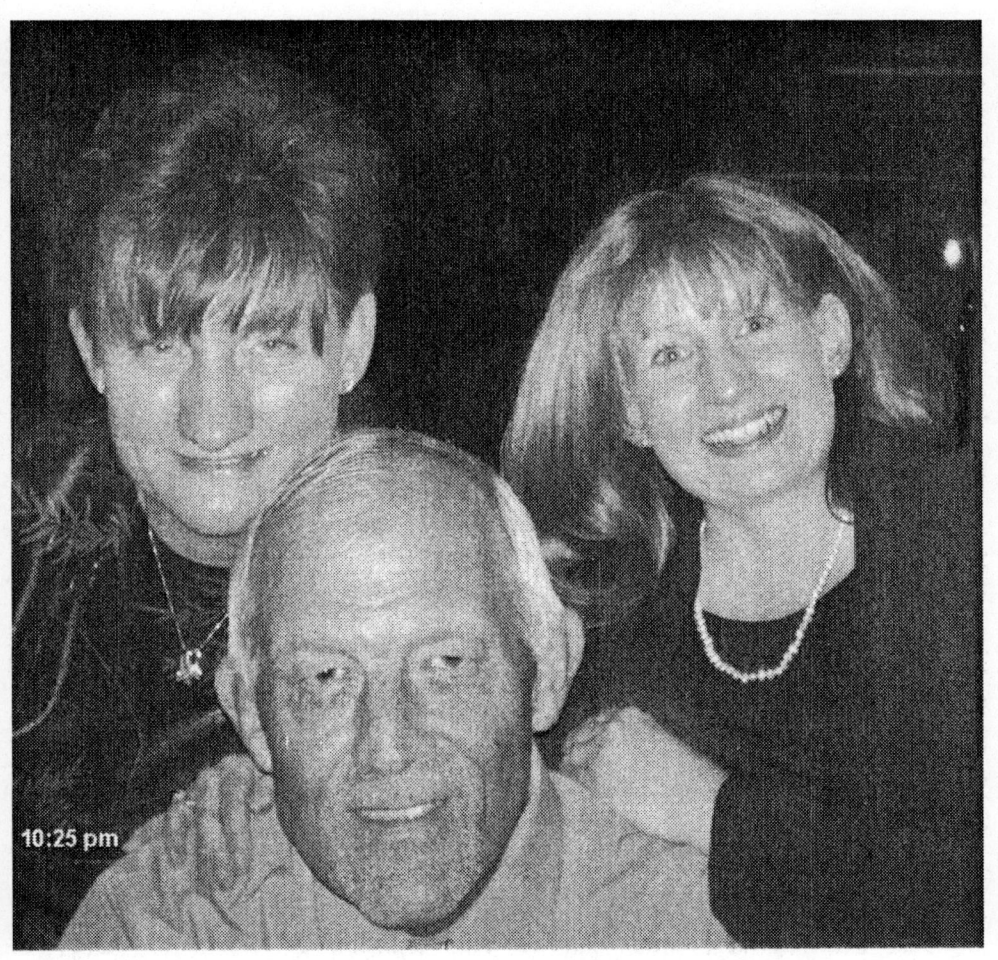

Family at a wedding, 2005

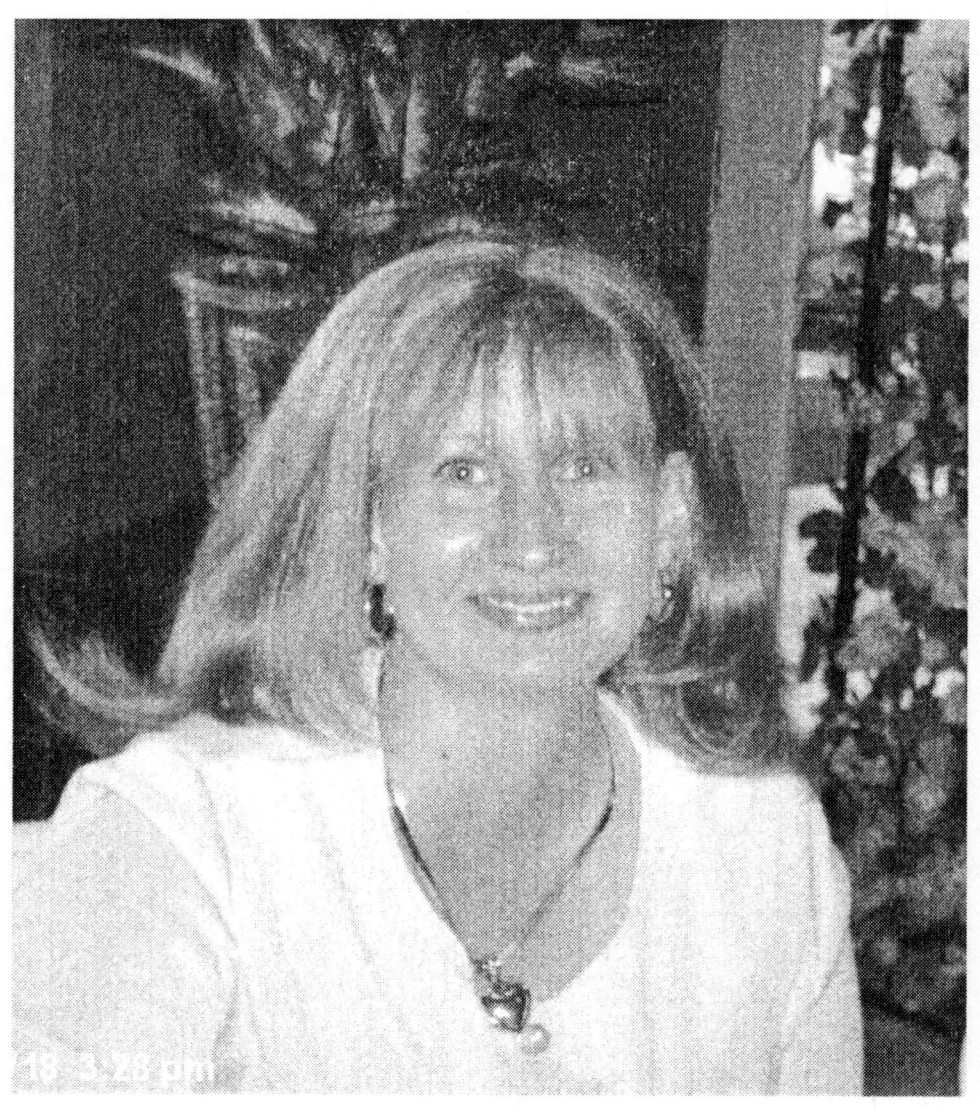

Ginger at another wedding, 2006

REFINED

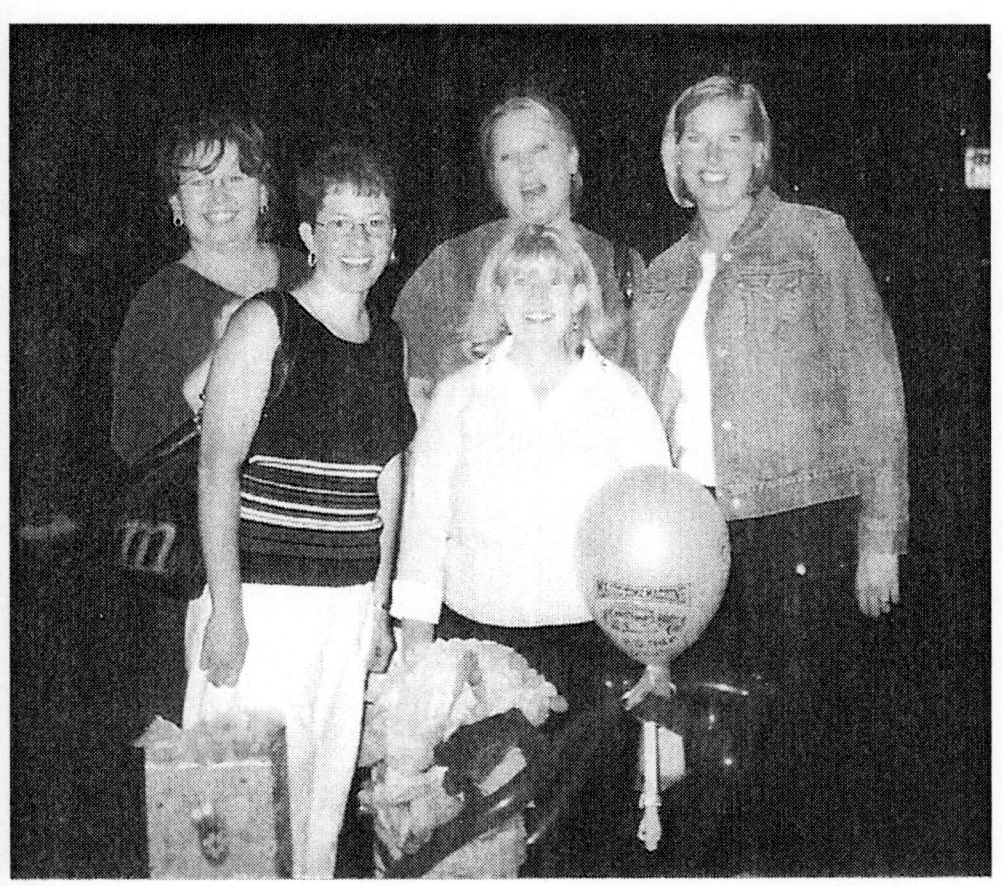

A part of the core support group, these young women have been together in the good and bad times. The bonds formed during Ginger's illness have remained strong. The experience has helped to shape the women they have become.

Chapter 6

The New Normal

January 1985

None of us was sad to see the end of 1984. We were hopeful that 1985 would be a better year. As we approached the new year, there was still old business to complete, so the scan and the removal of the temporary shunt was scheduled. January came, the scan was clear and the shunt could be removed. We would spend a couple of days in the hospital after the surgery. Relieved by the news that the tumor was gone, this surgery seemed minor when compared to all the other procedures. We officially entered the follow-up stage. Over the next years we would return to the clinic for evaluation and scans. Initially the appointments were every three months, then six months, then finally once a year. Ginger became a star in the clinic. She related well to the staff, both nurses and physicians, and they enjoyed her visits. She met their questions with honesty and spunk. She was recruited to start the St Paul fund raiser race in 1985. To the medical community she was a success story. To us and to the family of faith that had upheld her with their prayers, she was a miracle.

Children with cancer face day-to-day monumental challenges and there really should be a way to shield them from ignorance and insensitivity. It is not that people intentionally are uncaring or lack sensitivity. Fortunately, most people have not had personal experience with childhood cancer, so their ability to understand and relate is limited. Returning to school was a traumatic challenge for all of us. The first few weeks she attended half days. I would take her to school, return home and sit by the phone just in case she needed me. I thought that I had covered all the bases. I had spent time with the principal and the school nurse. I expected that the administration would prepare the teachers. But of course you can never prepare for all possible scenarios. The first week back in school there was an incident with the reading teacher. A stickler for rules, she demanded that Ginger remove the bandana she was wearing, since any head gear was against school policy. I only got bits and pieces of the interchange. Ginger was in tears, the teacher was humiliated, and this "momma bear" was ready to fight to protect her baby. The situation was resolved, and by the end of the year, student and teacher had formed a tight bond that lasted for years. This experience and others like it screams out for advocates to raise community education and awareness.

I returned to work when Ginger was able to return to full days at school and somehow we all made it through the semester. I am not sure how good I was at work, but it helped to focus on others and to keep busy. There was the school nurse, who spent a lot of days with Ginger on her lap in tears because of some heartless remark by a classmate or thoughtless comment of a teacher. She was fragile physically and emotionally. God surrounded her by protective friends and many wonderful teachers. She confronted school with the same conquering spirit she had faced each challenge. She would come home to be comforted and built up to daily face a world that had no understanding of how much the illness and its treatment had changed her. The experience had not only changed her, it changed her parents, too. None of us would ever be the same. It would be a long time before any of us would take any small blessing for granted.

Parenting doesn't come with an instruction manual and preadolescent girls seem to have specific rules of engagement. Saying no to a child with a life-threatening illness brings an overwhelming guilt. However, discipline is a necessary though difficult parenting task. In our one-child family we have always had a motto which we stuck with through recovery. Our child, like most American children, might very well be spoiled, but she would not be undisciplined. We set limits and where possible followed the approach of natural and logical consequences. Lest I sound hypocritically like the "perfect parent"—she rarely pushed the limits, so it made her adolescent years pretty easy. The most difficult task in returning to normalcy was that of letting go. The normal maternal instinct of overprotection was heightened, and it has taken years of practice to trust God to take care of the details.

Ginger's core group of friends must be credited for keeping her grounded and allowing her to be normal. Initially, they surrounded her and protected her. A teenager's worst fear is being different. Of course the hair loss was the most obvious difference. I remember being a youth sponsor for a mission trip. It was during that trip that I experienced the depth of commitment the group had to each other. As they were standing in line at Disneyland, the girls became aware of another group of girls who were staring at Ginger and whispering. Being accustomed to this kind of activity, she just ignored it and let it slide. Her friends on the other hand weren't inclined to let it go and took on the sensitivity training of the other group of girls, informing them that it was rude to stare at someone who had experienced cancer treatment. As they grew through the difficult teen years they remained close, challenged each other to grow spiritually, and held each other accountable. The greatest gift they gave her was the gift of acceptance. They were her friends on the good days and bad days. They allowed her to have meltdowns when the situation merited. She could just be herself, with or without hair, quiet or rowdy, happy or sad. The real friends were separated from the fair-weather ones and those who stuck were matured and blessed in the process.

The experience of cancer has a way of reordering priorities. When you feel that your time may be limited, it puts things into a new perspective. Initially, introspection is appropriate and necessary. What is really important and what gives meaning to relationships and life? There were activities that just didn't seem to matter much anymore. There is an internal struggle with the value of tomorrow. Confronted with the prospect of limited tomorrows, some things just aren't important. However, there is the hope that there may be many tomorrows—and given the fact that this child may indeed grow into an adult, school is still very important. Enjoying the moment and living every single day to its potential becomes priority number one. For several years following treatment we wore ourselves out trying to cram in as much living as possible. I was convinced that Ginger was trying to make up for lost time. However, at a point in her teen years, I finally came to the conclusion that being a person of many interests and activities was a trait she had inherited from me and not a consequence of any loss she might have felt. Finding the happy medium of living in the moment and preparing for the future remains one of life's greatest challenges

Chapter 7

Aftereffects

A Bad Hair Day Beats a No Hair Day, Any Day

Several years into her recovery, Ginger's junior high class would be given the assignment to write about their worst day. Ultimately, she wrote something less significant. She wasn't ready to write her story at that time. But she came home with the knowledge that most kids don't really know what a bad day is. "Tell me your worst day and I bet I can top it!" No hair has been a continuing problem. Most cancer survivors will grow new hair. That wasn't the case for Ginger. Accepting that the alopecia was permanent was a particularly difficult blow. Every time she looked in the mirror, she was reminded of what she had been through. It is sometimes hard to be gracious when others are complaining that their hair just won't behave. She'd trade anyone bad hair for no hair. Initially, wigs were ruled out as unnatural and uncomfortable. In her totally honest approach to life, she held the view "This is me. Take me or leave me." After researching the market, hairpieces have been the solution to looking natural. Years later she still has days when she expresses the desire that she could have her hair back. But on the good days her response is "You bet it's my hair; I paid lots of money for it!"

Why Is It So Hard?

Before medulloblastoma, school had always been easy for Ginger. She was a quick learner. After radiation, learning tasks became increasingly difficult. Math was particularly a challenge. She had difficulty focusing, but we persevered and her grades initially remained high. From the time she went back to school, I became her at-home tutor. We worked very hard at mastering the skills that she needed to succeed in the academic world. Her grades were average to above average. Most of the educators were relatively supportive, though because she now looked normal, it was hard to explain to them why there was a problem. She graduated from high school and made plans to go away to college. The radiation oncologist had warned us that there could be a drop in her intellectual capabilities and when algebra issues surfaced at college we sought out his counsel. When I asked about historical data for previous patients, he had none to give me. Only half of the children with Ginger's diagnosis had survived 10 years and of those none had gone to college. Ginger joined a study group and with the oncologist's help she was able to request un-timed testing for her math course. She completed the course with a "C." She was more proud of that "C" than of the other higher grades on her transcript. She completed a bachelors of arts degree in interdisciplinary studies and earned multiple state certifications in education. Her accomplishments are a great source of pride for her and for us as her parents because we know how hard she worked to obtain her education. More than a source of pride, these accomplishments are a testimony to God's miracles in her life. She was living against the odds and she was accomplishing much more than was expected by medical standards and statistics.

Why Me? Why Now?

After over twenty years as a childhood cancer survivor, the worst was over, or so one would think! Life was pretty normal. Ginger had been living independently for some time. She had been teaching in inner city Dallas for several years. She was preparing for continuing education classes. Just as suddenly as with the initial diagnosis, her world turned upside down again. We had been out to dinner that summer evening. She was working on our computer and was preparing to go home to her apartment. She began to experience strange symptoms, which we would later learn was a visual aura. She started describing things she was seeing to me and the situation quickly deteriorated. Kerry and I took her to the emergency room at Baylor, where she had a full-blown seizure, the first she had ever had. As Kerry and I sat in the waiting room, all the fear that we had experienced twenty years earlier returned. The leap to recurrence was our first thought. A C.T. scan revealed that scarring from one of her previous surgeries or perhaps the after effects of radiation was causing the problem. She spent the weekend in the hospital and underwent additional tests which confirmed the diagnosis. We were reassured that medication could control the seizures and that in time she would be able to resume her normal activities. Ecstatic we thought everything would be just fine and we would go back to our normal routine.

It proved to be somewhat more of a challenge than first indicated. It took months and several medications to find the right regimen for her. The new administration at the school where she was assigned was less than supportive and ultimately Ginger decided to take a medical leave of absence. She was very articulate about her condition. She would describe her mental status as feeling like she was living in a 12-story building with an elevator that only goes to the 8th floor. She was angry and disillusioned. Why would this surface now after so many years? This is a question that appears not to have a good answer. It has taken time and patience, but with determination and support she continues to work at overcoming yet another obstacle.

Socioeconomic Challenges

The after-cancer experience has included socioeconomic issues. Federal Law does have provisions to protect cancer survivors from losing insurance and from discrimination. However, in order to avoid pre-existing penalties, there can never be a lapse in insurance coverage. For Ginger this could have easily been a challenge. When she was out of work, she managed to maintain her insurance, though she went through all of her savings to do so. Loss of insurance means inability to pay for expensive medications as well as the necessary medical care. Some survivors have reported job discrimination because of their illnesses. Long-term effects of treatment can leave the survivor with deficits that affect their ability to pursue certain career paths.

Emotional and Social Issues

"Is September ever going to come and I won't feel this way?" I asked this question of one of my psychologist friends one evening when I was feeling particularly down. She replied, "Yes, but it will be a very long time." She was so right! For years I would begin to feel an unexplained sense of gloom and dread as we approached late August and early September. The first few anniversaries took me by surprise, but after some experience I learned to anticipate the time of year and planned something special to counteract the depression. Labor Day was Kerry's time. He loved to hunt, and we had an understanding that the weekend would be his time away. Early on Ginger and I began to plan a mother-daughter weekend. It became our weekend to connect, communicate and do the girly things we enjoyed and Dad tolerated.

Even though we could not have been more loved and supported by our friends and family, there was still a sense of isolation. There were times that I longed to meet someone who had been through the same challenges and survived. I would have loved to have seen a child who was on the other side of treatment and doing well. I felt as if no one really understood the fear and anxiety or the issues we were confronting. Worse than my sense of isolation was the emotional pain I watched my daughter endure. I tried my best to be in touch with her emotionally. She resisted any attempt to involve her in a support group. She gathered around her a close-knit group of friends who supported her. However, as supportive as they have been and continue to be, there is still no way they can really understand the depth of her experience. One of the most difficult emotions is the feeling of being different. All of us want to feel like we belong, and very few of us want to stand out in a negative way. The cancer experience puts you in a club you never wanted to join. It's an exclusive club, one which you can't and wouldn't want to invite your friends to be a member.

We call it the "pity party." You have these parties alone. No one else is invited and no one else comes. You recount all the reasons your life sucks! You cry because things aren't the way you want them to be! You talk to God and tell Him all the things you are feeling and all the things you have been through! You ask Him "Why?" "Why me?" "Why now?" "Why don't You help?" "What did I do to deserve this?" Sometimes a word from God will come in Bible study or quiet time or through a friend. Sometimes God is silent, but sometimes He wraps you in His love and says "I know." Other times you look inward or sometimes in the mirror and the answer becomes clear. Life is a gift! For as long as my life lasts, I will choose to live it in gratitude. I will find ways to share my experiences and my life in a way that brings glory to the God who gives me life and who sustains me.

Chapter 8

Celebrating Life

Remember when you were a kid. You counted the weeks until spring or summer vacation, the days until Christmas, the minutes each Friday afternoon until the weekend. I have always enjoyed celebrations. Holidays and birthdays have traditionally been major events in my life. I enjoy decorating for each season and each holiday. I look for occasions to have family gatherings. I am the family member or friend who jumps in and plans any celebratory event. I just love to be a part of making things special for the honoree. As much as I love Christmas, it really isn't my favorite holiday. I love Easter best of all. I love spring with its promise of new life and new beginnings. Driving along the roads seeing the Texas bluebonnets and other wild flowers carpet the hillsides reminds me to thank God for all the beauty that surrounds me. Every year I try planting flowers with a sense of hope that this year I'll be more successful as a gardener. And even if I don't succeed, it is pretty for a little while. Most of all I love Easter because it celebrates Christ's resurrection and the promise that life on earth is not all there is. Because of Easter we have the freedom to celebrate every day of life on earth and look forward to the promise of eternal life in heaven with Christ.

One of our most valuable coping mechanisms during treatment was celebrating small victories and small milestones. Every day became a celebration. Yeah! We made it through today, count down to the end of radiation, or whatever the current challenge might have been. During the first year following treatment we approached each holiday as though it might be the last one we would spend together. The net benefit of living life in that attitude is that we have had many all-out celebrations. When every day is viewed as an opportunity to celebrate life, little joys are heightened and little annoyances are minimized. The challenge is staying in a celebratory attitude. Each day life with its agitations has a way of clouding the joy we want to experience.

For the past three years Ginger, her life-long best friend, Frankie, and I have participated in American Cancer Society's Relay for Life. I love this event because it celebrates survivorship. The first time I observed the survivor's walk I was prepared to be emotional. I expected to cry as I watched my daughter round the track. However, that was not the emotion that overwhelmed me. As I stood with my team, I watched the many survivors as they walked the track in their purple shirts. The last woman across the line was an older woman walking with her son and daughter on either side. She was far behind the group of walkers. She could have easily sat down and no one would have thought less of her. But she kept on pushing herself with a spirit of determination to cross the finish line. It was a picture to me of the spirit of survivors. They keep on going when it would be easier to give up. They celebrate milestones along the way and they encourage others by their example. This is the spirit that inspires me to go to work every day and do my small part to make each patient's quality of life today the best it can be. To celebrate with them daily the victories that they choose to share with me. It is my honor to be a part of the lives of these courageous individuals and their families.

Spring of 2004 loomed as a landmark for Ginger. She was turning thirty. We began to ask how she wanted to celebrate her birthday. As with many women turning thirty, she would just as soon have skipped it. But having me as her mother ignoring birthdays really wasn't an option. However, I did remember the experience of turning thirty and promised to keep the celebration low key. Sometime during the spring, Ginger experienced one of those life altering "Aha!" moments. She had been doing some soul searching and was feeling guilty about her whiny attitude over turning thirty, being single, and whatever the issue of the day happened to be. She informed me that she had decided instead of moaning about the fact that she was turning thirty, she was turning it around and celebrating the fact that she was a twenty-year cancer survivor. Frankie and I jumped on that opportunity and decided to plan an all-out survivor celebration.

The survivor celebration was planned to be a surprise. We planned every detail. Kerry went on his yearly dove-hunting trip. Frankie, Ginger and I planned a weekend away, including shopping, dinner and a live show. By Sunday evening we had Ginger convinced that the weekend had been the celebration of her twenty-year anniversary. Her cousin, Amy, was assigned to keep her busy and away from my house on Monday, while Frankie and I decorated and prepared for the party. I was supposedly babysitting Amy's sons so that the girls could have some quality time together. Everything went off without a hitch. Many of the people who had held us together through her illness were there to celebrate this milestone. Surprise doesn't come close to describing her expression. She was completely overwhelmed. What a wonderful night! We celebrated that she was alive! We celebrated the person she is! Most of all we celebrated the miracles God has done in all of our lives. Each of us in our own way has grown spiritually because of the miracles that we experienced with Ginger. Seeing God work in her life has touched many lives. One card from a childhood friend said it best. "Your life is proof that God hears and answers children's prayers."

For me, just surviving has never been enough. Life is meant to be cherished and celebrated. God intends us to have an abundant life! In John 10:10, Jesus tells us, "The thief comes only to steal and kill and destroy; I have come that they may have life and have it abundantly." Another translation says "that they may have life and have it to the full." Abundance is defined as a great supply, having more than enough. That's what God wants for us—more that just enough, more than just existing. He has provided beauty in nature and a world of incredible wonders. He has blessed me with a wonderful family to love be loved in return. How dare I waste time and allow anything to steal my joy! Full is defined as occupying all of a given space. When my life is full of bitterness, anxiety, past hurts, fear, and anger there is less room for joy, peace, patience, and kindness. Each person has the choice—God's best, an abundant life, choosing to focus on the blessings, or the allowing the thief to choke out the best, getting us to settle for a life of simply surviving.

Chapter 9

The Present

    If someone had ever told me I would work as an oncology nurse, I would have said no way—no how—not me. There is a long list of reasons why I thought this would not be a good idea. I've been the care-giver, and I would get too emotionally involved. I would burn out quickly. It will be depressing. It would hurt too much too watch people I care about suffer and die. The list could go on and on. God has a sense of humor! Just tell Him that something can't happen! Over the past five years I have worked for Texas Oncology. What my patients have taught me and have given to me is far more than I could ever give to them. It has become my philosophy that I want to help them have the best quality of life possible for as long as possible. Many of the patients we see are long-term survivors and are living full lives. Each patient and each family has their own unique story. There are some common threads that bind us all together, but each individual brings to the experience something different and each one is special. Though busy and stressful, it is by far the most rewarding job I have ever had. God has a plan for me. He has used my experience to give me a heart for hurting patients as well as their family members. I am passionate about survivorship! My calling is to be an advocate for my daughter as well as other patients in the workplace, with the insurance companies, and anywhere I can raise public awareness of survivor issues. God has used my patients to teach me about courage and living life fully, and I am affirmed that He is using me to touch their lives.

    Kerry worked in industry throughout our early marriage, but changed careers in mid-life. He currently teaches high school. He loves teaching and is happy with the life-changing choice. God has a plan for him as well. Teaching is a calling, not for the faint hearted. The greatest reward comes when a student returns for a visit, or perhaps he meets them in the community and learns that they are succeeding. He has always had a gift for celebrating the present and letting aggravations go by the wayside.

We will celebrate our 38th wedding anniversary this June. Statistics indicate that marriages where there is a chronically ill child are more susceptible to divorce. One parent may devote so much time to the child that the marriage relationship is neglected. Our commitment to God, to the marriage and to each other has sustained us through the difficult times. I feel very blessed to be married to my best friend. Kerry's humor has diffused many difficult situations. Sharing the pain has forged a bond between us. I hope that we have years to grow old together. We are opposite in so many ways, with different temperaments, communication styles, and interests. The reality of our shared experience challenges us to live in the moment as much as possible and to find common ground.

Ginger feels a strong calling to work with children. She prefers to work with children one on one or in small groups, where she is able to see their progress. It is her strong desire to make a difference in the lives of the students she touches. While she isn't always patient with herself, she is very patient with small children and really enjoys the dimension they bring to her life. She lives independently, but visits us often. She turns watching sports on television into an interactive event as an involved spectator. Hockey is her current favorite sport. Go Stars! She is a movie buff, favoring the chick flicks. She will watch her favorites until many of the lines are committed to memory. She is one of the most giving individuals I know, choosing to support causes that benefit children. She especially loves Christmas. It has become her holiday tradition to shop for Toys for Tots or some other agency. Remembering her 10th Christmas, she never misses the opportunity to give back.

Cancer has changed our life perspective and philosophy. I would never have wished to experience cancer in our family. Since Ginger's illness, we have lost Kerry's dad to lung cancer, his mother to emphysema, and his sister to heart disease. Currently we are living with my dad's lung cancer and my step-dad's colon cancer. Each of these experiences has a pain and grief of its own. However, for me there has been nothing like the life-threatening illness of my child. It has made us the tightknit family that we are. Ginger will tell you that it has made her the woman that she is today. Her teacher was right—adversity does build character. And as the line in *Steel Magnolias* says "That which does not kill us, makes us stronger."

Chapter 10

The Future

If you could see into the future, would you *really* want to know? When I held my newborn daughter, would I have wanted to know the difficulties that her future held? Would knowing the challenges ahead of our family have changed the way we lived the first ten years? Absolutely! The fear and anxiety would have been crippling! Disciplining her would all but have been impossible for me. Could all that anxiety change the outcome? Not by my human efforts! Many times in scripture we are told fear not, don't fret, don't be anxious, don't worry about tomorrow. If God can control the universe, can I trust him to take care of my life and its problems big and small? Too often I have found that the things I worry about never happen. Before Ginger's illness, it would have never occurred to me to worry about a brain tumor. Bad things happen to everyone. Every person who lives on earth has a story, some more dramatic than others. God never promised us that we wouldn't have heartache and pain. In fact, to the contrary He tells us that in this world we will have trouble. The good news is that He is in control. In Matthew 6:34 Jesus gives us a direct admonition. "Therefore, do not worry about tomorrow, for tomorrow will worry about itself. Each day has enough trouble of its own."

Today is yesterday's tomorrow. What happened to all those yesterdays that became tomorrows? How did I spend them? Did I use them to ease someone else's hurt? Did I share an encouraging word? Was I too busy to listen? Was I too stressed to pay attention? Did I miss an opportunity to be God's hands in the world? These are the questions that haunt me. I have been given today. Tomorrow is not promised. Those people that touch my life may not cross my path again. I am the only person that has my exact experience. Kerry and Ginger have their own perspective on the same events. When I reflect on my day and realize that I missed opportunities, I am drained and conflicted. On the days that I follow my calling and make myself available, I realize that one person can make a difference. Those days are fulfilling and satisfying.

Organization and planning are essential to almost any successful event. Planning ahead is a way of being responsible for the resources that God has entrusted to us. There is a tension to find a balance between looking forward to the future and enjoying the present. The danger is that when so much time and effort is spent planning for the future, simply enjoying today gets lost in the process. God has a plan for His children. He knows me better than I know myself. He knows my strengths and my weaknesses, and He challenges me to let Him be glorified in both. The Bible refers to hope for the future. One of my favorite promises is Jeremiah 29:11 telling me that I indeed have a bright future. "For I know the plans I have for you, declares the Lord, plans to prosper you and not harm you, plans to give you a hope and a future." What a precious promise! No matter what my plan for my life is, I trust God to have a better plan. I just want to experience all He has in store for me.

Chapter 11

Lessons from the Cancer Experience

Life Is a Gift!

Before I was a mother, I prayed earnestly for a child. I wasn't sure that it would ever happen. When Ginger was born, I knew that her life was a precious gift to be treasured. After the cancer experience, the gift of her life became even more precious. I treasure the times we spend together. I treasure her friendship. I have learned to treasure my own life as a gift as well. I want it to be lived in a spirit of gratitude.

I Can Control Nothing!

For a control freak like me this is a very hard lesson to learn, one that I have to re-learn on a regular basis. Despite evidence to the contrary I seem to think I can fix things. I try to fix things for Ginger and for Kerry and ultimately drive the two of them nuts. Consistently, I have to return to my Father, give Him the mess I have made of things, and ask Him to do whatever it takes to make things right.. When I surrender the control of my life, I can live in peace and assurance that He is working things out for my best.

The Most Important Things in Life Are Not Things

We have been blessed with a lot of things, and it seems the more things you have, the more things you *need.* As I get older, I am realizing that the things I really need are few. The best times and the greatest memories don't involve things at all. Instead, it is spending time with family, sharing, playing and just being. The greatest pleasure for me today is feeling God's presence in Nature.

Friends and Family Are What Really Matters

When I think about the difficult times I have been through, I cannot imagine surviving those times without my family and my close friends. Lifelong friends prayed for us when we could not pray for ourselves. Friends supported us emotionally, spiritually and financially when we were not able to do it for ourselves. The bond forged by the experience of Ginger's illness made sisters of her friends. They became my daughters, and their parents became Ginger's parents. Because of these bonds, I know that we can count on each other in any of the crises of our lives.

Make Memories

Today is the only day I have. I will make it count. I take a lot of pictures, so that I have a visible reminder of the memories we make. There is something comfortable about keeping traditions, some things that we always do, like the breakfast casserole on Christmas morning. Traditions remind us of where we come from and help us feel grounded. The times spent playing cards and baking cookies or wishing I could have one more piece of Maw Maw's chocolate pie become the stories that are shared by the younger generations. The granddaughters sure wish that they had learned how to make that chocolate pie!

Memorize Scripture

In a crisis, focusing enough to read may be difficult if not impossible. In the darkest of times, scripture that I had memorized would come to me in the exact moment that I needed the assurance of its truth in my life.

Teach your children to "hide God's word in their hearts." It will carry them in difficult times and could very well help them to make wise decisions. Knowing what God says adds wisdom to decisions and comfort in the hardest of times.

People Have an Incredible Capacity for Giving

I learned that when there is a need, most people want to try to find a way to meet it. They passionately want to find a way to help, and they have a capacity to care deeply.

Allowing Others to Help You Blesses Both You and Them

It is often easier to give than to receive. Pride can stand in the way of accepting help. Refusing an offer of help robs not only the person who needs the help, but it robs the giver of a blessing.

Healing Is a Process

True healing begins when you are able to reach out to someone else who is hurting. About two years after her surgery, Ginger and I were asked to go and visit a young girl and her mother who were in the crisis of treatment. It was a difficult thing to do. Going back to the hospital was not easy. It brought back painful memories. I honestly don't know if we were able to help the other family or not as there was no ongoing contact. However, I know that when we were able to step out of the victim role and reach out to someone else, we moved into another level of healing. It was the first time we were able to allow our story to be used as an encouragement to someone else.

Career—Making a Difference, Not Just Making a Living

I have always felt that nursing was a calling for me. However, I have never considered myself a career woman. Today, I know I am doing exactly what God wants me to do. I will be open to His leadership for any future endeavors. For me, it is not about making money; it is about making a difference. I am learning daily what that means, because every day is a different challenge.

God Can Bring Beauty from All of Life's Experiences, Even Cancer

I believe with all sincerity that the loving God I serve does not will illness and pain in our lives. We live in a broken and fallen world. There is pain that is beyond our human understanding. With certainty I know that God can use the broken pieces of our lives, our hurts, our illnesses and bring good from them. I have a stronger faith in God and a closer walk with Him because of this experience. I have seen other people's lives touched and changed because of Ginger's story. Her life is evidence that God is still in the miracle business.

God Is Faithful

God promises us that He will be in the pits of our lives. When I could see nothing but darkness, He was in the darkness with me. When I couldn't pray, I found the promise in Romans 8:26 to be true, "the spirit prays for us with groanings too deep for words." When I was at the end of my rope, He reached down to me and assured me to take hold, He wasn't going to abandon me. In my spirit I could hear him say, "Hang on, child, I have you and I won't let go."

Prayer Changes Things

Praying may or may not change your situation. God may choose to miraculously heal. With all my heart, I believe He can and does heal this way in some cases. At other times, He uses the medical community to bring healing. The hardest of all to accept and understand are the times that death and heaven become the ultimate healing. No matter how healing comes, and though we may not get the outcome we desire, prayer changes our perspective from the finite to the eternal.

Chapter 12

Practicing the Presence of God

Nothing can separate us from the love of Christ. Life is hard. We live in a fallen world marred by all kinds of disasters. Times of crisis seem to make our dependence on God a necessity. When things are going along smoothly it is easy to feel self-reliant and put God in a box. But when events are beyond human control, when a miracle is needed, the focus on God becomes a priority. My story of cancer and its effect on our family ultimately is a story of relying on God. The times that I felt my human strength at its lowest were the times I felt the presence of God strongest. While Ginger's illness is one of the hardest trials I have faced, it is not the only problem I have had. I often have felt convicted that I have to have my back against the wall before I seek God earnestly. Growing spiritually is a discipline and I am still learning what that means in my life

Long commutes in heavy traffic are a stressful fact of most of our lives. However, rather than grousing about the traffic and delays, I have begun to use the time to reflect on the skies. God has used my recent commuting experience to teach me lessons in practicing His presence. As I drove to work one morning, I became aware of a bright ribbon of light connecting the front of my car to the sun. Stuck in traffic, I began to focus intently on the light. It was as if the light was a rope that connected me to the sun. Perhaps it was more like an umbilical cord that attached me to the light. As I began to reflect on God's presence in my life, I likened the sun to God, constant, always available. Like the big truck that broke my view of the light, sometimes our problems block our view of God. Sometimes it isn't something bad that gets in the way of our vision. Had that ribbon of light been there before? I suspect so. I just had never noticed it, because in my rush to get to work, I was focused on other things. In the same way the busyness of life can distract us from the presence of God in our lives. When I changed my direction, I lost sight of the light. The sun hadn't moved. The sun's ray still shone on my car, but my vision was focused in another direction. My walk with Christ is so like that. Some days my full attention is focused on Him and I am aware of His presence in everything that I do. Other days I go about my life as if I think I am in control, moving away from His presence. There is no overt evil present. I just am not aware of His presence in my life. God hasn't changed. He is the same today, yesterday and tomorrow. He is always there, reaching out to me. It is me that makes the difference. When I move away from Him, when I change my focus, I cheat myself out of the blessings He wants to give me.

The presence of the sun is one of those things easily taken for granted. It is a constant on which we have come to depend. On those days when the sun is bright with few clouds in the sky, I reach for my shades to block the brilliance of the light. I can not look directly at the sun for to do so would cause pain and possibly harm to my eyes. Much like that as I experience God revealing light on some area of my life that needs repentance, I am made uncomfortable and often have a difficult time facing Him directly. On days that are gloomy and overcast I can't see the sun, but I never question that it is there; I trust from experience that I will see the sunshine again. I also know from experience that growth cannot happen without the clouds and rain. The parallel to spiritual growth is painfully obvious. By far the most beautiful sunrises occur when the sun shines through the clouds. The reflection and the colors are brilliant and at times breathtaking. Like the sun, God is present even when I do not see Him. He is working in my life, even when I do not feel Him. His glory is revealed when I allow Him to work through my difficult circumstances and let His light shine through the clouds of my life.

Chapter 13

But What Do I Say? How Can I Help?

Often people will be at a loss for words when someone they care about is facing a loss or an illness. The most comforting thing you can do for someone who is hurting is to simply be there. Just knowing the support and love of family and friends is enough.

Some of the most comforting words shared with me were:

—Trust yourself. Gather the best information you can; make your decisions based on that information, and don't spend time looking back or second guessing yourself.
—I am here if you need me… to talk, to listen, or just to be here.
—I am praying for you.
—I love you.
—I hurt with you.
—I care that you are hurting.

If you want to help someone through the cancer experience:

Do:

—Be there.
—Share helpful, uplifting stories. Encourage. Be sensitive enough to know how and when sharing your story may be helpful.
—Send cards. They can be read and re-read and bring comfort in times when no one is around.

—Be normal. Normalcy is hard, but what is desired.
—Be yourself.
—Laugh if it is appropriate. Laughter is healing and can be a safety valve for pent-up emotions.
—Find ways to celebrate the present.
—Allow the patient and family to express their feelings, whatever they may be. They may experience the gambit of emotions and may change from moment to moment.
—Listen more and talk less.
—When you have the means to do so, meet a specific need. Acts of kindness large and small will be remembered for years in to come.
—Do household chores or provide someone to do housecleaning.
—Run errands.
—Provide meals that freeze in disposable containers.
—If you see something that needs to be done, do it.
—Babysit. Give the parents time to be alone as a couple.
—Be sensitive to clues that indicate unspoken needs.
—Hope.
—Pray for your friend and with them when appropriate.

Don't:

—Preach—Even great wisdom delivered at the wrong time can be more hurtful than helpful.
—Overstate the obvious.
—**Never** say, "I know just how you feel." No one really knows how another person feels in a specific situation.
—Talk about the patient as if they are not in the room.
—Act as if there is no hope.
—Act as if the person is dying or already dead.
—Feel like you need to fill the air with words.
—Tell a hurting person about your relative or friend who died from the same disease.
—Share your "horror stories" of treatment or disease.

—Offer unsolicited advice.
—Tell the person how they should feel.
—Give up hope.
—Expect God to work on your time table or to act in the way you want.

Scriptures to Strengthen and Heal a Hurting Life

In the same way, the spirit helps us in our weakness. We do not know what we ought to pray for, but the spirit himself intercedes for us with groans that words cannot express.
—Romans 8:26

The Lord is my shepherd, I shall not want.
He makes me lie down in green pastures,
He leads me beside quiet waters,
He restores my soul,
He guides me in paths of righteousness for his name's sake.
Even though I walk through the valley of the shadow of death,
I will fear no evil, for you are with me;
Your rod and your staff they comfort me.
You prepare a table before me in the presence of my enemies.
You anoint my head with oil;
My cup overflows.
Surely Goodness and love will follow me all the days of my life,
And I will dwell in the house of the Lord forever.
—Psalm 23

But those who hope in the Lord will renew their strength. They will soar on wings like eagles; they will run and not grow weary; they will walk and not faint.
—Isaiah 40:31

But now, this is what the Lord says—
He who created you, O Jacob,
He who formed you, O Israel:
Fear not, for I have redeemed you;
I have summoned you by name;
You are mine.
When you pass through the waters,
I will be with you;
And when you pass through the rivers, they will not sweep over you.
When you walk through the fire, you will not be burned:
The flames will not set you ablaze.
For I am the Lord, your God, the Holy One of Israel, your Savior;
 —Isaiah 43: 1-3

Have I not commanded you? Be strong and courageous. Do not be terrified; do not be discouraged, for the Lord your God will be with you wherever you go.
 —Joshua 1: 9

Trust in the Lord with all your heart and lean not on your own understanding; in all your ways acknowledge him, and he will make your paths straight.
 —Proverbs 3:5-6

And we know that in all things God works for the good of those who love him, who have been called according to his purpose.
 —Romans 8:28

For I know the plans I have for you," declares the Lord, "plans to prosper you and not to harm you, plans to give you hope and a future.
 —Jeremiah 29: 11

The Lord will fulfill his purpose for me; your love, O Lord, endures forever—do not abandon the work of your hands.
–Psalm 138:8

...being confident of this, that he who began a good work in you will carry it on to completion until the day of Christ Jesus.
–Philippians 1:6

Rejoice in the Lord always, I will say it again: Rejoice! Let your gentleness be evident to all. The Lord is near. Do not be anxious about anything, but in everything, by prayer and petition with thanksgiving, present your requests to God. And the peace of God, which transcends all understanding, will guard your hearts and your minds in Christ Jesus.
–Philippians 4: 4-7

I can do all things through Christ who gives me strength.
–Philippians 4:13

Be joyful always, pray continually, give thanks in all circumstances, for this is God's will for you in Christ Jesus...
May God himself, the God of peace sanctify you through and through. May your whole spirit, soul and body be kept blameless at the coming of our Lord Jesus Christ. The one who calls you is faithful and He will do it.
–I Thessalonians 5:16. 23-4

In the darkest days of Ginger's illness I found it very hard to concentrate enough to read much of anything. However verses that I had memorized would come to my mind at exactly the right time. Another way that scripture found its way to my conscious mind was on the many cards that arrived daily. I found comfort and healing in scripture. It was as if God was speaking directly to my soul. Some verses became a part of the hope to which I clung. God was and is in control of every situation. Despite my best efforts, I can't change the situation; I can only try to control the way I respond to it. He is with me every step of the way. He does not promise that things will be easy, just that he will be present. One of the dearest gifts I received was a copy of John Claypool's book *Tracks of a Fellow Struggler.* Isaiah 40:31 became my life line. Claypool, whose eight-year-old daughter died of cancer, wrote of God's grace. Some days will be soaring days of celebration; others will be days of running full of busy activity. Neither of those is appropriate at the bedside of a critically ill child. On those most difficult days, perhaps God's greatest gift is the grace which allows us to just put one foot in front of the other, to keep on keeping on. God promises to guide my decisions, and He has a plan for my future as well as the future of those I love. As long as I am alive and breathing, He continues to work in and through me, refining me, to complete His plan for me. Simply surviving is not enough. Being a survivor carries with it the responsibility to do something with the life God has allowed me to continue. Living life in an attitude of rejoicing, not anxiety, is not an easy choice, but certainly the healthiest. He promises us a peace beyond human understanding. God is faithful! If He said it, He will do it!